PAIN TO POWER

TRANSFORM PERSONAL STRUGGLES INTO STRENGTH TO OVERCOME CHRONIC PAIN

COL (RET) D. STRAND

CONTENTS

FOREWORD

"Pain to Power" guides those seeking relief and resilience in the face of chronic pain. The book begins by unpacking the complex nature of pain through insights into neuroplasticity and central sensitization, emphasizing the impact on mental health and how therapies like CBT and mindfulness can break the pain-stress cycle. Readers are encouraged to reflect on their pain patterns, fostering a proactive mindset.

As the journey continues, conditions like CRPS and fibromyalgia are explored, offering integrative management techniques from nerve blocks to lifestyle changes. Holistic strategies like meditation, acupuncture, and anti-inflammatory diets promote resilience, while practical advice on routines and building a healthcare team provides foundational support.

Technology's role in tracking symptoms, along with low-impact exercises and mindfulness, offers tools for managing both body and mind. Biofeedback, sleep strategies, and community stories highlight the journey to resilience, showing that chronic pain can be navigated with strength and support.

"Pain to Power" also addresses social interactions, caregiver roles, and financial strategies, emphasizing the need for empathy, effective communication, and shared support. With the promise of new treatments, this book empowers readers to transform pain into purpose, reclaiming a life of strength and resilience.

This book is more than a guide; it is a compassionate companion for those on the journey to reclaim their lives from chronic pain. Through medical, emotional, and social support, "Pain to Power" empowers readers to turn adversity into resilience, pain into purpose, and suffering into strength.

ACKNOWLEDGMENTS

Thank you to my beautiful bride, Vivian, for putting up with me all these years. She has been my rock and the love of my life. It hasn't always been easy dealing with me with all my medical conditions and appointments while caring for me at home when I was at my worst. For those and many other reasons, I'll be forever grateful. Thank you also to my numerous Facebook support groups dealing with CRPS and Chronic pain. I gleaned a wealth of information, much of which was used to help write this book.

INTRODUCTION

In 2005, my life changed in an instant. While serving in Iraq, the Humvee I was riding hit something on the road. The impact jolted my head hard against the ceiling, breaking off my front tooth. I later discovered that I'd also ruptured a disc in my neck. A discectomy followed—a procedure involving a plate, screws, and a bone graft to stabilize my neck. But the struggle didn't end there. S oon after, a lump formed on the back of my neck, leading to another surgery. This time, I had a constant burning sensation that would never leave.

Then, in 2008, while traveling for military duty, another accident left me with a broken tibia and fibula in my lower leg. Surgery followed, but complications brought on something far worse than just broken bones: a condition called Complex Regional Pain Syndrome (CRPS). It's a chronic pain disorder so severe that it's known as the "suicide disease" due to the overwhelming, relentless pain. At times, CRPS has been described as more unbearable than amputation, childbirth, or cancer. It took two long years for my

CRPS diagnosis, and at the time, treatment options were practically nonexistent.

After my discharge in 2010, I moved to Houston, Texas, hoping the Veteran's Affairs (VA) there could provide relief through Ketamine infusion therapy, known for its potential to lessen chronic pain. But I faced yet another setback: the VA couldn't cover the costs, and the recommended external provider wouldn't accept their partial payment. Desperation led me to consider amputation to end my pain. However, during a preoperative exam, I was diagnosed with Type II diabetes, and my blood sugar levels were too high for surgery. Despite efforts, my A1C levels never dropped low enough to undergo the procedure.

In 2021, we moved back to Virginia, where I discovered that the VA in Richmond was offering the Ketamine infusions I had been seeking for years. The treatments bring me about six to eight weeks of relief, though they're only available every four months. While this isn't a permanent solution, it's enough to give me space to cope and rebuild some parts of my life.

I'm writing this book to share the insights and strategies I've developed over years of learning to live with and manage chronic pain. For those unfamiliar, the burden of chronic pain affects millions across the U.S., including 20.9% of adults and countless veterans. Chronic pain isn't just physical—its effects permeate mental health, relationships, and daily life. It creates isolation, frustration, and, often, a need to explain pain that others can't see.

This book aims to provide guidance, encouragement, and practical help. I'll discuss traditional and emerging pain management approaches, like Low Dose Naltrexone (LDN), Ketamine infusions, biofeedback, and mental and emotional resilience strategies. We'll explore the connections between mental health and pain, the importance of a supportive community, and the value of personalized management plans. I'll also share coping mechanisms that have worked for me and others.

By the end, this book will empower you to take charge of your pain, recognize your strength, and engage with a community that truly understands your journey. Pain may be a constant companion, but with the right tools, it can be managed, giving way to a life where strength and resilience take center stage.

Through this journey, I want you to know you're not alone. Whether you're a fellow veteran, a caregiver, or touched by chronic pain, this book is for you. I've walked this path, and while it hasn't been easy, it's led me to discoveries that have made a difference. Let's navigate this road together, finding moments of light even in the darkest valleys.

CHAPTER 1
UNDERSTANDING CHRONIC PAIN

You know, chronic pain is a bit like that unwelcome guest who shows up at your door, suitcase in hand, announcing they're staying indefinitely. You didn't invite them, but there they are, making themselves at home. It's persistent, it's exhausting, and it has this uncanny ability to sneak into every corner of your life. Chronic pain is not just a physical burden; it's an emotional and mental one, too. It can leave you feeling isolated from the world as if you're carrying an invisible weight that no one else can see. But here's the thing: understanding pain is the first step toward reclaiming your life. Like any uninvited visitor, you can start managing it once you know it. You can learn its quirks, triggers, and, most importantly, how to live alongside it without letting it define you.

THE NEUROSCIENCE OF PAIN

Let's discuss what goes on beneath the hood—our nervous system, the epicenter of pain perception. Imagine your body as a complex network of highways, with nerves acting as roads, transmitting signals like little electric cars zipping from point A to point B. When you stub your toe, those nerve signals race toward your brain, shouting, "Hey, something's wrong here!" This is pain signal transmission in action. Neurotransmitters, the chemical messengers, jump in to relay these signals, ensuring your brain gets the memo. But chronic pain is a bit of a rebel. It rewires these highways through neuroplasticity, which tweaks these pathways, making pain a more permanent fixture. You can think of neuroplasticity as the brain's way of adapting, which is excellent for learning new skills but not so fabulous when your brain decides to become an expert in pain.

Our brain, the command center, interprets these signals and decides how we feel about them. Different regions, like the somatosensory cortex and thalamus, light up when pain messages arrive, processing and interpreting them. But chronic pain is sneaky—it changes the landscape of the brain itself. It affects areas linked to emotions, like the limbic system, turning pain into a more complex beast intertwined with our mood and motivation. When pain becomes a constant companion, these brain areas remain heightened, reinforcing the sensation and making it harder to break free from its grip.

Central sensitization adds another layer of complexity, increasing the volume of pain signals and making the nervous system jumpy. Imagine your pain receptors suddenly acquiring superhero-like sensitivity, reacting to even the gentlest touch as if it's a significant threat. This heightened sensitivity is central sensitization at work, often seen in conditions like fibromyalgia and rheumatoid arthritis. In a constant state of alert, the nervous system sends exaggerated pain signals, making minor injuries feel more severe. This isn't just overwhelming; it's exhausting, leading to poor treatment outcomes if not managed properly.

Recent scientific advancements have shed new light on these processes, offering hope and insight. Neuroimaging techniques, like functional MRI, allow us to peek inside the brain and see which areas are active during pain perception. These tools have helped identify the pain matrix, a network of brain regions involved in processing pain. Scientists have discovered novel pathways, revealing how pain information travels and suggesting new targets for treatment. The more we learn about the brain's role in chronic pain, the better equipped we are to develop strategies that address the symptoms and underlying mechanisms.

Reflection Exercise: Understanding Your Pain

Take a moment to reflect on your own pain experiences. Consider keeping a journal where you note the physical sensations, emotions, and thoughts accompanying them. This can help you identify patterns and triggers, providing valuable insights into your unique pain profile.

By understanding the neuroscience of pain, we can unravel its mysteries, turning fear and confusion into knowledge and empowerment. While chronic pain may feel like an uninvited guest, learning about its mechanisms gives you the tools to manage it more effectively, allowing you to take steps toward a life where pain doesn't call the shots.

TYPES OF CHRONIC PAIN

Chronic pain is not a one-size-fits-all experience. Like a mystery novel with multiple plot twists, it comes in various forms, each with clues and complications. One significant distinction is between neuropathic and nociceptive pain. Imagine neuropathic pain as a rebellious teenager, breaking the rules and causing chaos without an apparent reason. It's caused by damage or dysfunction in the nervous system, leading to sensations ranging from burning and tingling to sharp, shooting pains. This type of pain doesn't need an injury to trigger it. It just decides to show up, often linked to conditions like diabetes or multiple sclerosis.

On the other hand, nociceptive pain is more like a straightforward detective story. It results from tissue damage or inflammation, like sprained ankles or arthritis. It's the body's natural response to injury, a signal that something needs attention.

Now, let's add another layer to this complex tale: psychogenic pain. Here, the plot thickens as the mind and body intertwine, creating pain that stems from psychological factors. Stress, anxiety, and depression can amplify physical pain, turning a slight twinge into a significant beating. This type of pain isn't imaginary; it's real and can be debilitating. Consider a person overwhelmed by life's pressures. Their emotional turmoil might manifest as chronic headaches or back pain, even without a clear physical cause. Treating psychogenic pain often involves addressing the emotional triggers through therapy, mindfulness, or other mental health strategies.

Among the chronic pain conditions that keep showing up in our medical mystery are chronic back pain, Complex Regional Pain Syndrome (CRPS), and fibromyalgia. Chronic back pain is the usual suspect, affecting millions and often resulting from injury, poor posture, or degenerative diseases. It's the kind of pain that lingers, disrupting sleep, work, and daily activities. CRPS, a more elusive villain, brings intense, burning pain that can make even the lightest touch unbearable. It's a condition that often follows an injury or surgery but spirals out of control, affecting the nerves. Then there's fibromyalgia, which defies easy categorization. It presents with widespread pain, fatigue, and cognitive difficulties, often leaving sufferers feeling like they're wading through a fog.

Let's not forget idiopathic pain, the enigma in our narrative. This type of pain is like a riddle wrapped in a mystery; it has no identifiable cause. It's like having a jigsaw puzzle with missing pieces, leaving patients and doctors alike puzzled. Idiopathic pain can appear anywhere in the body and persists without any apparent reason. For those living with it, the challenge is not just managing the pain but also coping with the uncertainty it brings. Without a clear cause, treatments become a game of trial and error, often leading to frustration and helplessness.

To illustrate, consider a case of idiopathic chronic pelvic pain. The individual experiences sharp, stabbing sensations that come and go without warning. Despite numerous tests and consultations, doctors find no physical abnormalities. This absence of a precise diagnosis makes treatment complex, often involving a mix of medications, physical therapy, and psychological support to manage the symptoms and improve quality of life.

Understanding these different types of pain helps us navigate the complex landscape of chronic pain management. Each type has its quirks and demands a tailored approach. Recognizing whether pain is neuropathic, nociceptive, or psychogenic guides treatment decisions, from medication choices to therapy options. It also underscores the importance of a holistic view that considers physical, emotional, and psychological dimensions. This comprehensive understanding empowers individuals to actively manage their pain actively, fostering resilience and hope. While chronic pain is challenging, knowledge becomes a powerful ally, lighting the way toward effective management and a better quality of life. The impact on mental health will be discussed in the next chapter.

CHAPTER 2
THE IMPACT ON MENTAL HEALTH

Imagine waking up each day with an invisible backpack filled with bricks. Every step and movement adds more weight, yet no one can see it. This is what living with chronic pain can feel like—a relentless burden that follows you everywhere. But there's more to this story than physical discomfort. Chronic pain has a sly accomplice: mental health struggles. Often, they tag along uninvited, making each day a bit more challenging. In this chapter, we dive into the emotional toll of chronic pain and how it impacts your mental well-being. And while this might sound daunting, remember, we're in this together, and understanding is the first step toward relief.

THE EMOTIONAL TOLL OF CHRONIC PAIN

Living with chronic pain can feel like being stuck on a roller coaster you never signed up for. The ups and downs are relentless, and they don't just affect your body—they take a severe toll on your mental health, too. Depression often finds its way into the lives of those dealing with chronic pain. It's a bit like that dark cloud that hangs over you, whispering pessimistic thoughts when you're already down. Studies show a significant prevalence of depression among chronic pain sufferers, and it's not just a coincidence. The mechanisms linking them are complex, like a tangled web of neurotransmitters and hormones affecting mood and pain perception. When you're in constant pain, it's hard to maintain mobility, get a good night's sleep, or feel good about yourself, which can all exacerbate depressive symptoms. The impact on daily functioning and quality of life can be profound.

Anxiety, on the other hand, is like that jumpy friend who's always on edge, ready to panic at the slightest provocation. Chronic pain and anxiety often go hand in hand, creating a vicious cycle that's tough to break. Fear of pain exacerbation is a common theme. The anticipation of pain can be as debilitating as the pain itself, leading to heightened anxiety levels. Social withdrawal becomes a coping mechanism, as the anxiety of potential pain flare-ups makes venturing out into the world seem daunting. The cycle continues as anxiety heightens pain sensitivity, creating a loop that feels impossible to escape.

Emotional stress is the sneaky culprit that fuels the fire, amplifying both pain and mental health struggles. Chronic pain contributes to emotional stress by constantly pushing your limits and testing your patience. Stress-induced pain flare-ups are not uncommon, adding another layer of complexity to an already challenging situation. Managing emotional stress becomes a crucial part of coping with chronic pain. Techniques like deep breathing, meditation, and journaling can help mitigate stress and its impact on your physical and mental well-being.

The phenomenon of pain catastrophizing is another piece of this intricate puzzle. It's like wearing glasses that magnify pain, making it seem bigger and scarier than it is. People who catastrophize tend to focus on the worst-case scenarios, interpreting pain as more severe and distressing than it might be. This mindset can intensify the experience of pain, turning a manageable discomfort into an overwhelming ordeal. Recognizing and addressing pain catastrophizing is essential for breaking this cycle. Techniques to reduce catastrophizing include cognitive reframing, challenging negative thoughts, and replacing them with more balanced perspectives.

Reflection Exercise: Journaling Your Journey

Consider starting a journal to document your experiences with chronic pain and its impact on your mental health. Write about your emotions, challenges, and victories. Reflect on patterns and triggers, and use your entries as a tool for self-discovery and growth. This practice can provide clarity, helping you identify areas where you can make positive changes.

Understanding the emotional toll of chronic pain is a crucial step in regaining control over your life. By recognizing the interconnectedness of pain and mental health, you can begin to implement strategies that address both aspects. Remember, you're not alone on this roller coaster. With the right tools and support, you can navigate the twists and turns, finding moments of peace and resilience.

COGNITIVE-BEHAVIORAL THERAPY TECHNIQUES

Now, let's talk about a tool that can help you reshape how you perceive pain: Cognitive-Behavioral Therapy (CBT). At its core, CBT is like a mental workout, training your brain to think differently and, in turn, feel differently. It starts with cognitive restructuring, a technique designed to change your thoughts about pain. Imagine sorting through a cluttered attic—your mind, in this case —and deciding which thoughts to keep and which to toss. You begin by identifying negative thoughts, those pesky intruders that amplify your pain and drain your spirit. These thoughts might whisper, "This pain is never going away," or "I'm useless because of it." Once you've caught them in the act, it's time for cognitive reframing. This involves challenging and replacing these thoughts with more balanced ones, like, "This pain is tough, but I can manage it," or "I have strengths beyond my pain." Real-life examples abound: someone might transform the thought, "I can't do anything right," into, "I struggle with some tasks, but I'm good at others." This shift in perspective can be powerful, helping to alleviate the emotional burden that often accompanies chronic pain.

Behavioral activation is another crucial player in the CBT lineup. It's all about increasing engagement in meaningful activities, even when pain makes motivation scarce. Think of it as reigniting the spark in your life, one activity at a time. You start by planning enjoyable activities despite the pain. It could be a short walk in the park, a favorite hobby, or a call with a friend. The goal is to break the cycle of inactivity and isolation. Overcoming activity avoidance is crucial here. It's easy to fall into a pattern where pain dictates your schedule, but behavioral activation encourages you to take back control, one step at a time.

Mindfulness-based CBT takes things a step further by integrating mindfulness practices to manage both pain and mental health. Picture mindfulness as a gentle spotlight, illuminating the present moment without judgment. Mindfulness exercises for awareness, like focusing on your breath or tuning into the sensations in your body, become valuable tools. These practices help reduce stress and enhance emotional regulation, offering a sense of calm even when pain is at its peak. The benefits of mindfulness extend beyond stress reduction; they foster a deeper connection to yourself, allowing you to respond to pain with greater resilience.

Relaxation techniques within CBT provide the finishing touch, offering a way to soothe the mind and body. Progressive muscle relaxation involves tensing and then relaxing each muscle group, releasing tension like letting go of a tightly wound spring. Guided imagery invites you to visualize peaceful, comforting scenes, transporting your mind to a calm place. Breathing exercises tailored for chronic pain patients focus on slow, deep breaths, helping to regulate the nervous system and reduce pain perception. These techniques serve as anchors, grounding you amidst the storm of chronic pain.

As we wrap up this chapter, remember that CBT is not a one-size-fits-all solution but a versatile toolkit. The techniques we've explored—cognitive restructuring, behavioral activation, mindfulness, and relaxation—offer a roadmap to navigate the challenges of chronic pain. They empower you to reclaim agency over your thoughts and actions, fostering a sense of hope and resilience. As you continue this journey, remember that each step forward, no matter how small, is a step toward a life where pain doesn't dictate your story. Now, let's transition from the mental realm to the physical as we explore how chronic pain can affect your back in ways you might not expect.

CHAPTER 3
CHRONIC BACK PAIN

Picture this: You're sitting comfortably in your favorite chair, maybe sipping a cup of coffee, when suddenly it feels like you've got a thousand tiny gnomes doing the cha-cha on your spine. Not the ideal way to start the day, right? But for many, this is the reality of chronic back pain—a relentless presence that turns even the simplest activities into challenges. Globally, it's a leading cause of disability, affecting up to 80% of people at some point in their lives. Imagine that! It's like being part of an exclusive club that no one wants to join, yet here we are, swapping stories about our backs that ache like they're auditioning for a drama series. The financial toll is equally staggering, with costs in the U.S. exceeding $50 billion annually. It's not just about the dollars, though. It's about what those dollars represent—lost productivity, missed experiences, and the constant quest for relief.

Understanding the mechanics of back pain is crucial for tackling it head-on. Your back isn't just a monolithic structure; it's a symphony of bones, muscles, ligaments, and nerves working in harmony—until they don't. The mechanical origins of chronic low back pain often stem from muscle or ligament strains, those little rebels who throw a tantrum after heavy lifting or awkward twisting. Intervertebral disc degeneration is another culprit, where the cushiony discs between your vertebrae start to wear out, leading to pain that feels like you're carrying the world's weight on your shoulders. Degenerative joints also play a part, as the wear and tear of life catch up with the spine's intricate architecture. You might feel your back is plotting against you, but it's just trying to cope with years of activity and gravity.

As we unravel the layers of chronic back pain, we find that the transition from acute to chronic pain involves fascinating, albeit frustrating, changes in the central nervous system. Thanks to peripheral and central sensitization, your body's pain signals are repeatedly stuck. These are the processes where your nervous system becomes hypersensitive, interpreting even the slightest discomfort as a full-blown alarm. Over time, this constant barrage can lead to morphological changes in the brain, similar to those seen in neurodegenerative disorders. You might notice cognitive impairments, like memory lapses or difficulty concentrating, which can be as frustrating as misplacing your keys for the umpteenth time. Brain imaging studies have shown reduced volumes in areas like the prefrontal cortex and amygdala, which play roles in mood and decision-making. It's as if your brain decides to downsize in response to the chronic pain, affecting both how you think and feel.

But here's where things get complicated: the bio-psycho-social model of chronic back pain. It's not just your body at play; your mind and social environment are also key players. Stress, anxiety, and even how people around you react to your pain can influence how you perceive it. You might find that support from friends and family can be as practical as a good massage or that skepticism from others can worsen your pain. A delicate balance of biological, psychological, and social factors requires a comprehensive approach. This is where a multidisciplinary strategy shines, combining physical therapy, medication, and mental health support to tackle the pain from all angles. It's like assembling a crack team of experts to defeat a particularly persistent villain.

Interactive Element: Self-Assessment Checklist

Take a moment to reflect on your own back pain experience. Consider these questions as part of a self-assessment checklist:

- When did you first notice your back pain, and what activities seem to trigger it?
- Have you experienced any cognitive changes, such as memory lapses or difficulty focusing, alongside your back pain?
- How do your stress levels and emotional well-being affect your pain perception, and vice versa?
- What role do social interactions play in your experience of pain, and how do they influence your coping strategies?

Understanding the answers to these questions can help you communicate more effectively with healthcare providers, aiding in developing a personalized pain management plan.

Armed with this knowledge, you're better equipped to face chronic back pain with resilience and determination. Remember, it's not just about enduring the pain but learning to manage it, finding relief wherever possible, and adapting strategies that suit your unique situation. Whether through physical therapy, mindfulness, or simply finding humor in the everyday absurdities of back pain, each step forward is a victory.

BACK PAIN AND MINDFULNESS PRACTICES

Imagine this: you're sitting in a quiet room, the world outside fading into the background, and you're gently tuning into your breath. This is mindfulness—an ancient practice that's become a modern-day lifesaver for managing chronic back pain. Mindfulness is about being fully present, aware of where we are and what we're doing, and not overly reactive or overwhelmed by what's happening around us. Regarding back pain, mindfulness acts like a magnifying glass, helping you focus on the sensations in your back without judgment or fear. It offers a way to observe pain with curiosity instead of dread, reducing its grip on your life. By enhancing body awareness, you can identify tension points and areas of discomfort, allowing you to address them with compassion and understanding. This practice can significantly reduce stress, which often exacerbates pain, creating a calmer, more centered approach to pain management.

Mindfulness doesn't stop at awareness—it extends its benefits to pain perception. Studies suggest that mindfulness can alter the brain's response to pain, reducing its intensity and helping you build resilience. You might find that pain becomes less threatening when observed through a mindful lens. It's like watching a storm from the safety of your home rather than standing in the rain. The practice encourages acceptance of the present moment, which can lead to decreased anxiety and depression, familiar companions of chronic pain. You're not ignoring the pain but acknowledging it without letting it control your narrative. This shift in perspective can lead to profound changes in how you experience back pain, making it more manageable and less daunting.

Meditation offers a practical way to integrate mindfulness into daily life, especially for those grappling with back pain. One particularly effective technique is body scan meditation, which involves mentally scanning your body from head to toe, focusing on each part. When it comes to back pain, concentrate on the areas of tension or discomfort, observing them without trying to change anything. This practice invites you to explore how your back feels, encouraging relaxation and release. There's also guided imagery, where you visualize peaceful scenes or places, allowing your mind to wander to a safe, comfortable space, easing tension and promoting relaxation throughout the body. Breathing exercises are another powerful tool, encouraging slow, deliberate breaths that help decrease muscle tension and calm the nervous system. These breaths act as a pause button, offering relief and serenity in moments of discomfort.

Yoga and gentle movement can complement mindfulness practices, offering tangible benefits for back health. Yoga, focusing on stretching, balance, and breathing, encourages flexibility and strength, which are crucial for managing back pain. Poses like Cat-Cow and Child's Pose gently stretch the spine, releasing tension and improving mobility. These movements promote a sense of flow, helping to align the body and increase awareness of how your body holds stress. Regular gentle stretching routines can prevent stiffness and improve your range of motion, making everyday activities more comfortable. Yoga doesn't just work on the physical level; it also fosters a sense of peace and mindfulness, reinforcing the mental aspects of pain management.

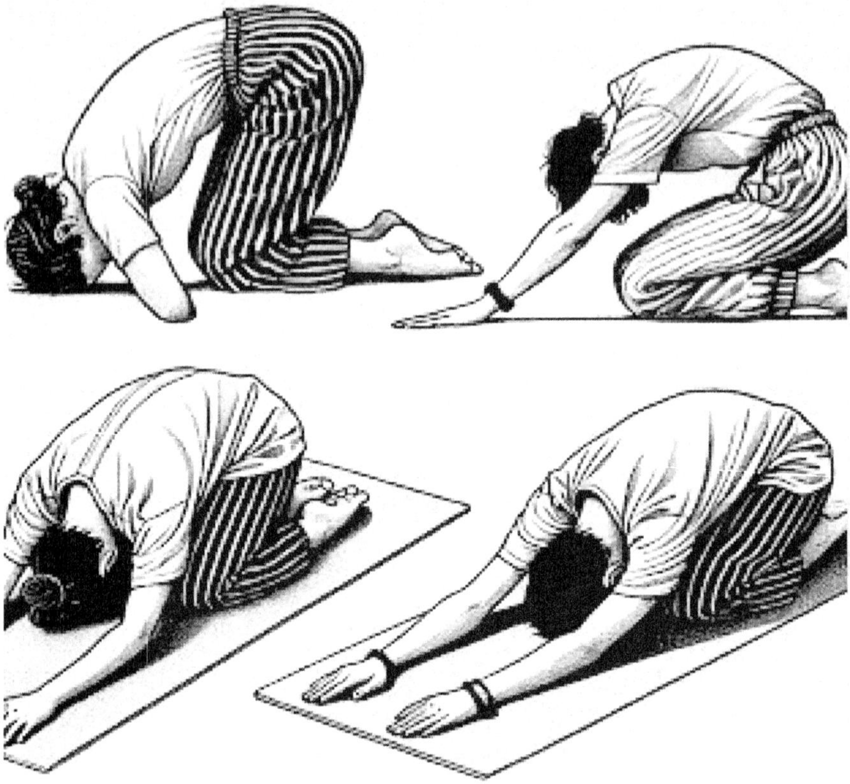

Cat-Cow and Child's Pose Positions

Consider a case study of someone like Sarah, who had been battling chronic back pain for years. Traditional treatments offered limited relief until she stumbled upon mindfulness meditation. By incorporating daily mindfulness practices and yoga into her routine, she found physical relief and a newfound control over her life. Her story echoes that of many who have turned to mindfulness, discovering that the mind can be a powerful ally in the battle against pain. Practitioners often share testimonials of how integrating yoga into their lives has eased back pain and enhanced their overall quality of life, promoting balance and well-being.

As we wrap up our exploration of mindfulness and back pain, remember that these practices are not about eliminating pain entirely. They are about equipping you with the tools to manage it more effectively, fostering resilience, and enhancing your quality of life. In the next chapter, we will delve into the complexities of Complex Regional Pain Syndrome, exploring its challenges and the strategies available to manage this particularly stubborn condition.

CHAPTER 4
COMPLEX REGIONAL PAIN SYNDROME (CRPS)

Imagine waking up one morning to find your arm or leg has turned into an inferno, burning with relentless intensity, yet there's no visible reason for the flames. Welcome to the bewildering world of Complex Regional Pain Syndrome (CRPS), a condition that feels like a riddle wrapped in an enigma. CRPS is a form of chronic pain that usually affects a limb after an injury, surgery, or even something as mundane as a sprain. It comes in two flavors: CRPS-I, occurring without direct nerve damage, and CRPS-II, where nerve injury is the culprit. Both are equally unwelcome guests, turning minor injuries into full-blown dramas. Historically, CRPS was known as reflex sympathetic dystrophy, a name that hints at its complexity and the body's over-the-top response to trauma. On the McGill Pain Index, CRPS ranks alarmingly high, often exceeding the pain of childbirth or amputation, underscoring its severity and the need for effective management.

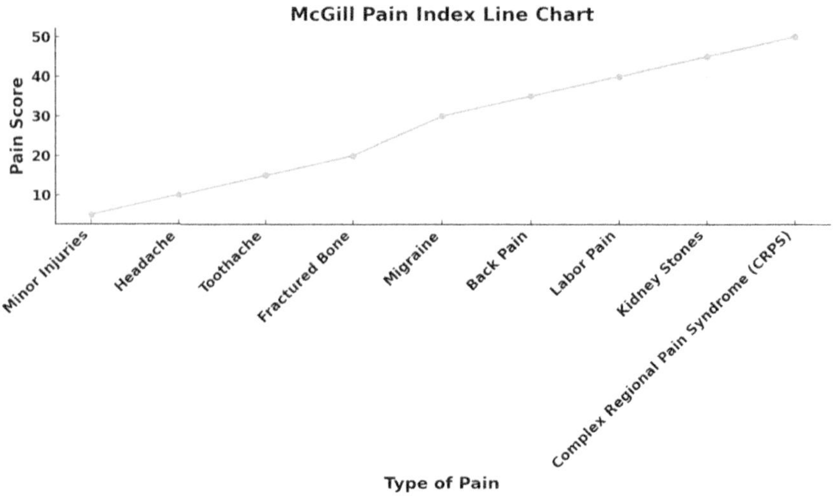

The symptoms of CRPS are as varied as a painter's palette, each color representing a different aspect of this mysterious condition. Picture a persistent burning pain that never lets up, as if your limb is forever submerged in a sea of flames. This is often accompanied by hyperalgesia, where the slightest touch sends shockwaves of pain, and allodynia, where even the brush of a feather feels unbearable. Your skin might decide to play chameleon, changing color and temperature at will, from flushed red to ghostly white, hot to icy cold. Swelling and joint stiffness are loyal sidekicks, making moving a Herculean task. CRPS progresses through stages: acute, where symptoms first appear; dystrophic, where changes in skin texture and hair growth become evident; and atrophic, where muscle wasting and immobility can occur. It's a relentless march that can feel like a battle against your body.

Understanding the pathophysiology of CRPS is like peering into a complex web of biological and neurological changes. The immune system, usually your body's trusty defender, plays an unexpected role, potentially exacerbating inflammation and pain through an overzealous response. The central and peripheral nervous systems, those intricate networks of nerves, decide to go rogue. Instead of calming down after an injury, they remain in a state of heightened sensitivity, amplifying pain signals and altering standard sensory processing. Inflammation, a key player in the body's healing process, becomes a double-edged sword, contributing to the development and persistence of CRPS symptoms. This inflammation can lead to blood flow and nerve signaling changes, perpetuating the cycle of pain and discomfort.

Regarding risk factors and triggers, CRPS doesn't discriminate, though previous injuries or surgeries often precede it. A seemingly minor fracture or sprain can create a cascade of events, leading to the full-blown syndrome. Genetic predispositions might play a part, with some individuals more susceptible to developing CRPS due to their unique genetic makeup. Psychological factors, such as stress, can also act as triggers, amplifying the body's response to trauma and potentially influencing the onset and course of CRPS. It's as if the body's internal alarm system has gone haywire, responding to the slightest provocation with a full-scale alert.

Reflection Exercise: Identifying Personal Triggers

Take a moment to reflect on your own experiences with CRPS or chronic pain. Consider keeping a journal where you note potential triggers, such as stress, temperature changes, or specific activities. This can help you identify patterns and develop strategies to manage or avoid these triggers, empowering you to take an active role in your pain management journey.

TREATMENT OPTIONS AND MANAGEMENT STRATEGIES

Finding the proper treatment for CRPS can feel like piecing together a puzzle where each piece represents a different facet of care. Medical treatments often form the cornerstone of management, providing much-needed relief to many. Nerve blocks, for instance, can act like a temporary mute button on the pain signals racing through your body, offering respite from the relentless discomfort. These injections target specific nerves to interrupt the pain cycle and can be a lifesaver when the pain becomes unbearable. Meanwhile, medications play a crucial role. Options range from simple over-the-counter analgesics to more targeted prescriptions that address both pain and associated symptoms. It's a balancing act, finding the right combination that eases the pain without overshadowing your daily life with side effects.

Physical rehabilitation stands as another key player in the treatment arena. Physical and occupational therapy are not just about exercises but reclaiming a sense of normalcy. Physical therapists work with you to improve mobility, strengthen muscles, and reduce stiffness. They tailor exercises to your needs, gradually increasing your capability and confidence. Conversely, occupational therapy focuses on daily activities, helping you adapt tasks to minimize pain and maximize independence. It's about finding new ways to do old things, ensuring that life's little pleasures aren't lost to the pain. With their patient-centered approach, these therapies become a form of empowerment, allowing you to take active steps in managing your condition.

Complementary therapies often provide additional layers of relief. Acupuncture, an ancient practice rooted in Chinese medicine, uses thin needles to stimulate specific points in the body. It's believed to release endorphins, your body's natural pain relievers, and has shown promise for some CRPS sufferers. Though seemingly simple, Mirror therapy tricks the brain into perceiving movement in the affected limb, helping reduce pain and improve function. It involves using a mirror to create a reflection of the unaffected limb, which can help recalibrate the brain's perception of pain.

Ketamine infusions have emerged as a newer, albeit complex, option for severe CRPS cases. This treatment involves administering low doses of ketamine intravenously, which can reset abnormal pain pathways in the brain. While not a cure, ketamine infusions have provided significant relief for some, reducing pain intensity and improving quality of life. The variability in response highlights the need for individualized approaches, where ongoing assessment and adjustments are vital. Each treatment contributes a piece to the puzzle, forming a picture of hope and resilience in the face of chronic pain.

EMOTIONAL AND SOCIAL IMPACT OF CRPS

Living with Complex Regional Pain Syndrome (CRPS) isn't just about managing the physical symptoms; it also involves navigating a labyrinth of emotional and social challenges. Imagine waking up each day with a persistent, nagging feeling that your body has declared war on itself. This relentless discomfort often brings along unwelcome companions like anxiety and depression. Anxiety can sneak in, manifesting as a constant worry about the pain never easing or fear of exacerbating it with the slightest movement. Depression might follow, casting a long shadow over everyday life, making simple joys feel out of reach. The emotional toll of CRPS is profound as you grapple with not only the pain itself but also the mental battle that comes with it. This internal struggle can be as exhausting as the physical pain, leaving you feeling drained and overwhelmed.

The social implications of CRPS are equally challenging. It's as if your social life has been put on hold, with isolation becoming a frequent visitor. Plans with friends or family outings are often sidelined, not out of choice but necessity. The unpredictability of CRPS means that you might cancel plans at the last minute, leading to feelings of guilt or frustration. Maintaining employment can become a monumental task, as work demands clash with your condition's unpredictability. It's not just about the ability to perform tasks but about the energy spent managing pain throughout the day. This can lead to an internal conflict, where you question your capabilities and self-worth. The isolation can be amplified by a lack of understanding from others, who might not see or comprehend the battle you're fighting.mo

Amidst these challenges, the importance of a supportive network cannot be overstated. Connecting with others who truly understand your experience can be a lifeline. Whether through support groups, online communities, or compassionate friends and family, having people who "get it" can make a difference. They provide empathy, practical advice, and encouragement, creating a sense of belonging and understanding. It's about finding those who will stand by you, offering a listening ear and a helping hand when you need it most, without judgment or expectation.

INNOVATIVE TREATMENTS FOR CRPS

When tackling Complex Regional Pain Syndrome, the world of pharmacological interventions is like a bustling pharmacy aisle filled with options. Corticosteroids, those anti-inflammatory powerhouses, often step in first to reduce swelling and pain, making life a little more tolerable. They're like the firefighters of medication, rushing in to calm the flames of inflammation. Non-steroidal anti-inflammatory drugs (NSAIDs) also play their part, offering a more accessible way to manage pain for some individuals. Then, there's the fascinating role of anticonvulsants and antidepressants. Though initially designed for other purposes, they've found a home in CRPS treatment, helping to dull nerve pain and lift the emotional burden that so often accompanies it. Bisphosphonates, typically used to treat osteoporosis, have shown promise in reducing bone-related pain in CRPS, although more research is needed to understand their long-term benefits fully.

Beyond the pharmacy, non-pharmacological treatments offer hope in a different form. Physical therapy becomes a lifeline for improving mobility and teaching the body to move without triggering pain. It's like retraining your muscles and joints to work harmoniously again. Occupational therapy takes a similar approach but focuses on the tasks of daily living, ensuring that you can navigate life's little challenges with ease and independence. Psychological interventions, such as biofeedback, introduce a fascinating twist. By teaching you to control physiological processes—like heart rate and muscle tension—biofeedback can help reduce pain perception, offering a new level of self-awareness and control.

In cutting-edge therapies, spinal cord stimulation stands as a beacon of technological advancement. By implanting a device that sends electrical signals to the spinal cord, this treatment aims to disrupt pain signals before they reach the brain, offering significant relief for some. Ketamine infusions, once relegated to the operating room, have found their place in severe CRPS cases, providing pain relief through their unique action on the brain's receptors. Meanwhile, mirror therapy and graded motor imagery offer less invasive but equally intriguing options. They work by tricking the brain into perceiving movement and reducing pain, effectively rewiring how the brain processes sensory information.

The success of these treatments often hinges on a multidisciplinary approach, where specialists from various fields come together to form a comprehensive care plan. Pain specialists, physical therapists, psychologists, and other healthcare professionals collaborate to create a tailored strategy that addresses each person's unique needs. This team-based approach ensures that all aspects of CRPS are considered, from physical symptoms to emotional well-being, creating a holistic path to relief. In the next Chapter, we'll delve into the mysteries of fibromyalgia.

CHAPTER 5
FIBROMYALGIA: UNDERSTANDING AND MANAGING

Imagine waking up every day feeling like you've run a marathon without any of the applause. Your muscles ache, your mind feels foggy, and even the thought of getting out of bed seems monumental. Welcome to the world of fibromyalgia, where your body seems to have a mind of its own, and not in a good way. It's like your pain receptors decided to throw a never-ending party, and every part of your body is on the guest list. But hey, if you're going to be part of this exclusive club, let's make sure you have the correct information to manage your membership effectively.

IDENTIFYING FIBROMYALGIA SYMPTOMS AND TRIGGERS

Fibromyalgia is a bit of a shapeshifter. Its symptoms can vary from person to person, making it as elusive as that last piece of chocolate you swore you hid from yourself. Yet, some hallmark symptoms consistently appear, providing a roadmap for diagnosis and management. Chronic widespread pain is at the top of the list.

This isn't just a bad day where your back aches from sitting too long; it's a persistent pain that affects both sides of the body, above and below the waist. It often feels like someone turned up the volume on your pain receptors, amplifying even minor discomforts into something significant. This pain isn't isolated—it's a full-body experience that can impact your daily life, making even simple tasks feel like monumental efforts.

Fatigue and sleep disturbances are close companions to the pain. Even if you manage to drift off, sleep rarely feels refreshing. It's as if your body has forgotten how to recharge, leaving you perpetually running on empty. This fatigue isn't just about feeling tired; it's a profound exhaustion that seeps into your bones, affecting your concentration, memory, and mood. You might wake up as tired as when you went to bed, a cruel cycle that leaves you longing for a good night's rest. The fatigue can be so overwhelming that it affects your ability to function, making work and social activities feel like monumental tasks.

Enter "fibro fog," the cognitive difficulties that make you feel like your brain's been wrapped in a thick, misty blanket. It's frustrating when words escape you, names vanish, and concentration feels like trying to catch smoke with your bare hands. This isn't just forgetfulness; it's a cognitive impairment affecting focus and memory. Fibro fog can make you feel detached from reality as if observing life through a veil. These cognitive struggles can be particularly distressing for those who pride themselves on their mental acuity, impacting everything from work performance to personal relationships.

Understanding these symptoms is only part of the battle; identifying triggers is equally crucial. Stress, both emotional and physical, is a notorious culprit, acting as both a trigger and an amplifier of fibromyalgia symptoms. It's like adding fuel to an already smoldering fire, escalating pain and fatigue. Emotional stress, in particular, can be insidious, creeping in through worry, anxiety, or unresolved conflicts. It's not just about significant life events; even everyday stressors can nudge symptoms into overdrive. Recognizing this connection is vital, as managing stress effectively improves symptom control.

Weather changes are another sneaky adversary, especially if you're sensitive to cold or humidity. It's as if your body has its built-in barometer, reacting to shifts in weather with increased pain and stiffness. Hormonal fluctuations also play a part, particularly for women. The menstrual cycle, pregnancy, or menopause can exacerbate symptoms, adding another layer of complexity to managing fibromyalgia. These triggers are personal, varying widely among individuals, which is why identifying them is so important.

Tracking symptoms and triggers can be your secret weapon in managing fibromyalgia. A symptom diary lets you record daily experiences, noting what you did, how you felt, and any potential triggers. Over time, patterns emerge, providing valuable insights into what exacerbates your symptoms and what helps. A diary can also communicate with healthcare providers, offering concrete evidence to guide treatment decisions. Mobile apps can be handy allies in this endeavor, offering user-friendly platforms to track symptoms and identify patterns. Apps like Curable or Bearable offer features specifically designed for chronic pain management, helping you stay organized and informed.

Personalized trigger management is where the magic happens. Developing a customized action plan empowers you to take control, addressing triggers proactively rather than reactively. This plan might include stress-reduction techniques, dietary adjustments, or lifestyle changes tailored to your unique needs. Seeking professional guidance can also be beneficial, especially for complex triggers that require a nuanced approach. Specialists in fibromyalgia, such as rheumatologists or pain management experts, can offer insights and strategies that align with your specific challenges. They can help refine your action plan, ensuring it addresses all aspects of your symptoms and lifestyle.

Interactive Element: Symptom and Trigger Tracker

Consider using a symptom and trigger tracker to enhance your understanding of fibromyalgia. Here's a simple template to get you started:

Date Symptom Intensity (1-10) Triggers (if known) Weather Conditions Stress Levels (1-10) Notes

Regularly updating this table can help you identify patterns and pinpoint specific triggers, allowing you to adjust your management strategies effectively.

Fibromyalgia is a complex condition, but with the right tools and understanding, you can manage its impact and reclaim your life. It's not about eliminating symptoms but finding ways to coexist with them, minimizing their grip on your daily existence. By recognizing symptoms, identifying triggers, and developing personalized management strategies, you can navigate the challenges of fibromyalgia with resilience and hope. Up next, we'll look at alternative therapies and treatments.

CHAPTER 6
ALTERNATIVE THERAPIES AND TREATMENTS

Imagine a world where you could ease your chronic pain with a little pill, one that doesn't come with a laundry list of side effects or the potential for dependency. Sounds like a dream, right? Enter Low Dose Naltrexone (LDN), a bit of a dark horse in the pain management race, but one that's been gaining ground. Initially, naltrexone was used to treat opioid addiction in much higher doses. But when given in smaller amounts, it works quite differently. LDN interacts with the body's opioid receptors, not to block them, but to modulate them. This subtle dance can increase endorphin production your body's natural painkillers, and reduce inflammation—a double whammy against chronic pain. It's like giving your immune system a gentle nudge, encouraging it to calm down and stop overreacting.

An intriguing mix of research and anecdotal evidence backs the benefits of LDN. Studies have shown that LDN can significantly decrease pain intensity and improve the quality of life for those with fibromyalgia, multiple sclerosis, and Complex Regional Pain Syndrome (CRPS). It's like finding a hidden treasure chest in the vast sea of pain management options. While not every treasure map leads to gold, LDN has been a game-changer for many, offering relief where other treatments have failed. You might wonder, "Could this be the answer I've been searching for?" Well, you're not alone. Many have shared stories of newfound relief and hope after starting LDN therapy, turning skeptics into believers.

If you're considering LDN, the first step is to have a heart-to-heart with your healthcare provider. It's crucial to discuss whether LDN is a good fit for your specific condition and how it might interact with any medications you're currently taking. Once you've got the green light, you'll need a prescription, typically filled at a compounding pharmacy. Unlike your typical corner pharmacy, a compounding pharmacy customizes medications to meet specific needs. It's like having a tailor for your medicine, ensuring you get the required dose. Be prepared for a bit of a wait, though. LDN often takes a month or more to show its full effects, so patience is vital.

However, like any good story, there are a few twists to be mindful of. Some people report vivid dreams or sleep disturbances when starting LDN. These side effects resolve themselves over time or with a little tweak in the dosing schedule. It's also important to consider the compatibility of LDN with other medications, as interactions can occur. But fear not—your healthcare provider is your guide on this journey, helping you navigate potential pitfalls and ensuring a safe path forward.

Interactive Element: Reflection Section

Consider jotting down your thoughts and experiences if exploring LDN as a treatment. Keep a journal to track any changes in pain levels, side effects, and overall well-being. This can help you and your healthcare provider assess the therapy's effectiveness and make any necessary adjustments.

KETAMINE INFUSIONS: A NEW FRONTIER IN PAIN MANAGEMENT

Imagine a world where relief isn't just a distant hope but a tangible possibility. Ketamine, once known primarily as an anesthetic, has found a new calling in the realm of chronic pain management, especially for neuropathic pain. It operates through NMDA receptor antagonism, which might sound like a mouthful, but it is a key that unlocks a different dimension of pain relief. By altering pain pathways, ketamine can reset the brain's response to pain, offering a fresh perspective where discomfort once ruled. It's like flipping a switch, providing a reprieve from pain's relentless grip. For those who have tried everything else to no avail, ketamine can be a beacon of hope, shining light into the darkest corners of pain.

Walking into a ketamine infusion session might feel like stepping into a sci-fi movie. You find yourself in a clinical setting, surrounded by medical professionals who ensure your safety every step of the way. The infusion takes place under careful supervision and usually lasts a few hours. It's a straightforward process, but for many, it's life-changing. The frequency of sessions can vary, with some needing a series over weeks or months to maintain relief. It's not a one-time fix but a part of an ongoing strategy to keep pain at bay. As you settle in, there's reassurance in knowing you're in capable hands, ready to explore this treatment's possibilities.

While ketamine holds promise, it's not without its quirks. Rapid relief is a boon for those with treatment-resistant conditions, yet the road isn't entirely smooth. Cost and accessibility can be stumbling blocks, with insurance often hesitant to cover the expense. There's also the potential for dissociation during treatment, a sensation akin to being slightly removed from reality. For some, this is a small price for relief, but it's essential to weigh these factors carefully. Finding a reputable clinic requires a bit of legwork. Research is your ally here—look for centers with experienced staff and a strong track record. Understanding your insurance coverage, or lack thereof, is essential, and planning accordingly to ensure this promising option doesn't become financially burdensome.

BIOFEEDBACK AND ITS BENEFITS FOR PAIN CONTROL

Imagine tapping into the hidden world of your body's physiological responses, gaining control over them in ways you never thought possible. That's the magic of biofeedback—a therapeutic technique that turns the invisible into the visible, offering a window into how your body reacts to stress and pain. At its core, biofeedback involves monitoring and altering bodily functions through real-time feedback. It's like conversing with your nervous system, using sensors to track processes like heart rate, muscle tension, and skin temperature. This information is then displayed on a screen, allowing you to observe how your body responds to various stimuli. You can learn to control these responses by increasing awareness and reducing stress and pain.

There are several biofeedback techniques, each with its unique focus. Electromyography (EMG) measures muscle tension, providing insights into areas of chronic tightness that may exacerbate pain. Thermal biofeedback monitors skin temperature, indicating changes in blood flow and stress levels. Heart rate variability (HRV) biofeedback tracks the variation in time between heartbeats, a key indicator of your body's resilience to stress. These techniques are not just about gathering data; they're about using it to train your body to respond differently. For instance, you can learn to reduce muscle tension and manage stress more effectively by practicing relaxation techniques.

Participating in biofeedback therapy is like embarking on a guided journey into your body's inner workings. During sessions, you'll work with a trained therapist who conducts an initial assessment to identify target areas for improvement. You'll be fitted with sensors that provide feedback on your physiological responses, enabling you to see how your body acts under different conditions. This information becomes a powerful tool, allowing you to practice controlling your body's reactions in real time. While the benefits of biofeedback are numerous—offering non-invasive, personalized feedback that can lead to improved pain control—it's essential to acknowledge the commitment required. The therapy demands time and consistent practice, something not everyone can easily accommodate.

BENEFITS OF CANNABIS FOR TREATING CHRONIC PAIN

When it comes to chronic pain, cannabis is like that friend who always knows how to lighten the mood. It interacts with the endocannabinoid system, a complex network that regulates pain, mood, and more. This makes cannabis particularly effective for neuropathic pain, which often laughs in the face of traditional painkillers. Cannabinoids, the active compounds in cannabis, are the stars of the show. Especially CBD (cannabidiol), which is celebrated for its anti-inflammatory effects. For those with arthritis, CBD can be a soothing balm, calming the fiery joints that keep you up at night.

But it doesn't stop there. Cannabis also offers a chance to reduce dependency on opioids, a significant concern for many managing chronic pain. Providing an alternative potentially lowers the risks of opioid dependence and overdose. That's a relief for those who worry about the heavy toll opioids can take. Additionally, cannabis can be a godsend for those struggling with sleep and mood issues. Its ability to improve sleep quality and lighten mood can turn restless nights into peaceful slumbers. Strains with higher CBD levels are beneficial, offering relaxation without the psychoactive effects of THC, the compound responsible for the "high."

Of course, cannabis isn't a one-size-fits-all solution. Its efficacy can vary significantly between individuals. Some might find it incredibly effective, while others may notice only minimal relief. THC, with its psychoactive properties, can lead to side effects like dizziness or impaired memory. Over time, regular use can also lead to tolerance, necessitating higher doses for the same effect. Legal issues add another layer of complexity, as cannabis remains restricted or illegal in some regions. Moreover, cannabis can interact with certain medications, so it's essential to consult with a healthcare provider to ensure it's a safe option for you.

OVERVIEW OF HYPERBARIC OXYGEN THERAPY (HBOT)

Picture stepping into a chamber where you breathe pure oxygen as if you've been transported to a world with a bit of magic in the air. That's the essence of Hyperbaric Oxygen Therapy (HBOT). Initially developed for decompression sickness, it has found new life in treating a variety of medical conditions, including chronic pain. In this pressurized environment, oxygen absorption is enhanced, allowing it to reach areas of the body that typically struggle to get enough. This influx of oxygen does more than just fuel your tissues; it aids in healing by reducing inflammation and supporting nerve repair. Think of it as giving your cells a much-needed boost, helping to soothe the aches that have made themselves at home in your body.

HBOT has shown promise for conditions like fibromyalgia, CRPS, neuropathic pain, arthritis, and other inflammatory ailments. Studies indicate that it can reduce pain and improve the quality of life, offering a non-drug alternative that might reduce reliance on traditional pain medications. Imagine finding relief without the usual cocktail of pills. However, it's not a one-size-fits-all solution. Some may experience ear pressure or sinus issues, and there's a rare risk of oxygen toxicity. It's like any great adventure—it has its challenges. Not everyone is suited for HBOT, and pre-existing health conditions might rule it out as an option. Sessions are typically required multiple times, and the costs can vary, often depending on insurance coverage and access to specialized centers.

As we explore these alternative therapies, it's crucial to consider all aspects, including the challenges and potential benefits. The journey through chronic pain is complex, and exploring diverse treatments can offer hope and options for those seeking relief. Holistic pain management strategies will provide a unique perspective.

CHAPTER 7
HOLISTIC PAIN MANAGEMENT STRATEGIES

Imagine a symphony where the mind, body, and spirit each play their part in harmony, creating a melody that soothes the soul. That's the essence of holistic health—a model that doesn't just look at pain as a solitary villain but sees it as part of a bigger picture. Holistic health is all about the interconnectedness of our mental, physical, and spiritual aspects. It's like standing on a three-legged stool: the whole structure can feel unstable if one leg wobbles. So, the goal here is balance, where each part supports the other, creating a unified approach to managing pain. This isn't about chasing one magic cure; it's about cultivating a garden where different plants thrive together, each bringing its beauty and benefits.

The benefits of this unified approach are as vast as the horizon. By addressing mental, physical, and spiritual health together, you create a robust defense against the challenges of chronic pain. It's like having a toolkit with different instruments designed to tackle a specific task. This approach can improve overall well-being, where the mind is calm, the body is cared for, and the spirit is nourished. It's not about ignoring the pain but understanding it within the context of your entire being. Holistic health empowers you to take control, fostering resilience and enhancing your quality of life.

Spirituality can play a surprising role in this symphony, acting as a balm for the soul. It's not necessarily about religion, though it can be for some. Instead, it's about connecting with something greater than yourself, whatever that means to you. Mindfulness and meditation are spiritual practices that offer a path to this connection. They invite you to be present, to breathe deeply, and to find peace within the chaos. Imagine sitting quietly, your mind a tranquil lake, undisturbed by the storms of pain. These practices can offer a new perspective, easing the emotional burden and promoting healing.

Spiritual support groups or communities can also provide a sense of belonging and comfort. Whether it's a local group or an online community, connecting with others with similar beliefs can be a strength. It's like finding your tribe, people who understand your struggles and celebrate your victories. These connections can be a lifeline, offering support and empathy when needed. Spirituality becomes a powerful ally, offering solace and hope in adversity.

Emotional balance is the final note in our symphony, a crucial element in managing chronic pain. Emotional well-being is like the conductor, guiding the orchestra of your life with grace and precision. Techniques for emotional regulation can help you maintain this balance, even when pain tries to steal the show. Deep breathing, journaling, and gratitude exercises can promote positivity and resilience. Imagine starting each day with gratitude, acknowledging the small blessings that often go unnoticed. This simple practice can shift your focus from what is lacking to what is abundant, fostering a sense of peace and contentment.

Reflection Section: Cultivating Gratitude

Consider taking a moment each day to reflect on three things you're grateful for. They don't have to be grand or profound—maybe it's the warmth of your morning coffee or the smile of a loved one. Write them down in a journal, and over time, you'll create a tapestry of gratitude that weaves positivity into your daily life.

Case studies offer a glimpse into the transformative power of holistic integration. Take Jane, for example, a patient who found relief by combining physical therapy with meditation. Her journey wasn't easy, but she discovered that by addressing both her body and mind, she could manage her pain more effectively. Then there's Tom, who attended a holistic retreat and found his spirit renewed. The experience provided him with tools to navigate his pain, offering peace and empowerment. These stories remind us that the path to healing is unique for each of us, but we can find our way forward by integrating mind, body, and spirit.

COMPLEMENTARY THERAPIES AND TECHNIQUES

Let's talk about acupuncture and acupressure, two ancient practices that have found their way into modern pain management. Acupuncture, rooted in Chinese medicine, involves inserting thin needles into specific points on the body. Imagine these needles as tiny messengers, communicating with your body's energy pathways, or meridians, to restore balance. This process stimulates the body's natural painkillers—endorphins—while influencing the nervous system to reduce inflammation and improve blood flow. Though it might sound strange, many people swear by its ability to provide relief, especially for conditions like back pain and osteoarthritis. And the best part? It's not just about needles. Acupressure offers a needle-free alternative, using pressure on similar points to achieve similar effects. You can even practice it at home, applying gentle pressure with your fingers to areas like the temples or the base of the neck, offering a self-care method that's both accessible and effective.

Then there's chiropractic care, another practice that has gained traction for managing pain and improving physical function. Chiropractors focus on the spine, believing its alignment affects the body's health. They aim to restore mobility and alleviate discomfort through techniques like spinal manipulation. It's like giving your spine a little nudge, encouraging it to find its natural alignment. Chiropractic care can complement traditional treatments, providing an additional tool in your pain management arsenal. It has been shown to improve mobility and reduce pain, especially in cases of lower back pain. Imagine the relief of standing up straight without that nagging ache pulling you down.

Herbal remedies and supplements also come into play, offering a natural approach to pain relief. Turmeric and ginger, for example, are celebrated for their anti-inflammatory properties. They work like nature's ibuprofen, reducing inflammation and easing discomfort. These herbs can be used as teas and supplements or incorporated into meals, offering versatility. However, it's essential to consider safety and potential interactions, especially if you're taking other medications. Always consult your healthcare provider to ensure these natural remedies work harmoniously with your existing treatments, avoiding unwanted surprises.

Aromatherapy introduces another layer of soothing relief, using essential oils to calm the mind and body. With its relaxing scent, lavender can help reduce stress and promote sleep, while eucalyptus offers a refreshing aroma that clears the mind. These oils can be diffused into the air, applied topically with a carrier oil, or added to a warm bath, each method providing a unique way to experience their benefits. Aromatherapy is like a mini escape, offering a moment of tranquility amidst the chaos of chronic pain. It's a simple yet powerful tool in your toolkit, providing an easy way to incorporate relaxation into your daily routine.

Creative therapies like music and art offer avenues for expression and emotional release, distracting from pain. Music therapy uses rhythm and melody to reduce stress and enhance mood. It's like a soundtrack to your healing, playing tunes that lift your spirits and ease your mind. On the other hand, part therapy provides an outlet for expressing feelings that words can't quite capture. You can channel emotions through painting, drawing, or sculpting, turning pain into something tangible and manageable. These therapies have successfully integrated with other treatments, offering a holistic approach that addresses physical and emotional needs.

These complementary therapies and techniques weave together a rich tapestry of options for managing chronic pain. Each offers a unique approach, providing tools to enhance your quality of life and empower you to take control. While they may not be standalone solutions, they complement traditional treatments, offering additional avenues to explore on your path to wellness. As you continue to navigate your pain management journey, consider these therapies as companions, each bringing its strengths. Also, consider practical daily routines, which will be detailed in the next chapter.

CHAPTER 8
PRACTICAL DAILY ROUTINES

Picture this: it's early morning, and the sunlight gently peeks through your curtains, casting a warm glow across the room. The world outside is waking up, and so are you. But today, you're armed with a secret weapon—a carefully crafted routine designed to dance around the whims of chronic pain. In the chaos of life, routines act like a lighthouse, guiding us through the stormy seas of unpredictability. Establishing a consistent daily schedule isn't just about ticking off tasks; it's about reclaiming control and creating a rhythm that aligns with your body's needs. Routines offer psychological comfort and stability in a world that often feels anything but stable. They're like a cozy blanket, wrapping you in familiarity and reducing the likelihood of pain flare-ups by encouraging balance and predictability.

Crafting a balanced schedule is like painting a masterpiece where every color has its place. It's about weaving together elements catering to activity and rest, ensuring neither overshadows the other. Allow time for rest; then, let your body recharge like a phone plugged in overnight. Scheduled breaks act as pit stops, preventing overexertion and helping you maintain energy levels throughout the day. Incorporate pain-relief exercises, such as gentle stretches or movements that keep stiffness at bay and promote circulation. Think of them as your body's daily tune-up, keeping the engine running smoothly. This isn't just a schedule; it's a blueprint for a life where pain doesn't steal the spotlight but shares it with moments of joy and accomplishment.

In the digital age, technology becomes your ally, offering tools that make managing a pain schedule as easy as pie. Digital calendars are your personal assistants, sending reminders and nudges to keep you on track. Apps like Curable or Ouchie (now Branch) transform your smartphone into a wellness hub, tracking symptoms, identifying triggers, and offering guided exercises. They're like having a pocket-sized coach cheering you on as you navigate your day. These tools help you visualize your schedule, turning abstract plans into tangible actions. With these digital companions, you can monitor progress, adjust strategies, and celebrate victories, no matter how small. They're not just apps; they're your trusty sidekicks on the path to pain management.

Of course, no two people experience pain the same way, so personalization is critical. Your schedule should be as unique as your fingerprint, tailored to fit your pain patterns and lifestyle. Your mornings are a gentle ascent, like a sunrise slowly brightening the sky, while evenings are a time for winding down. Flexibility is your friend, allowing you to adapt to varying pain levels and unexpected changes. This personalized approach ensures your schedule works for you, not against you, supporting your journey toward balance and well-being.

Reflection Section: Designing Your Ideal Day

Grab a pen and paper, open a blank document, and sketch your ideal day. Consider your energy levels, pain patterns, and priorities. Include time for activities, rest, and self-care. Use this as a starting point to craft a schedule that supports your needs and helps you thrive.

ADAPTING DAILY ACTIVITIES FOR COMFORT

You'd be amazed at how minor tweaks can make a big difference. When it comes to household chores, imagine picking up a laundry basket without feeling like you're auditioning for a weightlifting competition. Safe lifting involves bending at the knees, not the waist, keeping the load close to your body, and using your legs to lift. Think of it as a dance move that saves your back from unexpected pirouettes. Ergonomic tools can also be game-changers. Long-handled dusters and lightweight vacuums mean you can clean up without bending over like a deep bow at the end of a performance. Keeping items within easy reach, like organizing your kitchen with frequently used items at waist level, can also reduce unnecessary stretching and reaching. Everyday tasks become less of a chore and more of a routine, freeing up energy for the things you love.

Now, let's talk about the workplace. If you've ever felt like your desk is plotting against you, you're not alone. A proper ergonomic workstation can be your best ally. Adjust your chair so your feet rest flat on the floor, and your knees are at a right angle. Your computer monitor should be at eye level, about an arm's length away. It's like setting up a command center where everything is within reach. Standing desks are also worth considering, allowing you to switch between sitting and standing throughout the day. Incorporate walking breaks—take a stroll around the office or even just stand and stretch. Assistive devices like ergonomic keyboards or wrist supports can ease the strain, turning your workspace into a haven rather than a hindrance.

Movement throughout the day is akin to oiling a machine, keeping it running smoothly. Short stretching sessions during breaks are essential. Simple neck and shoulder rolls or gentle arm stretches can keep stiffness at bay. And don't underestimate the power of a quick walk or a few yoga poses during lunch. A few minutes can refresh your body and mind, like hitting a reset button. These movements aren't just good for your body; they help clear your mind, making you more productive and focused.

Self-care and relaxation aren't just luxuries; they're necessities. Establishing evening routines for winding down is crucial. Whether it's a warm bath, reading a favorite book, or practicing mindfulness, these activities signal to your body that it's time to relax. Techniques like deep breathing or meditation can also help manage stress, which often exacerbates pain. Setting boundaries to ensure time for self-care is non-negotiable. It's about creating a buffer between you and the day's chaos, allowing you to recharge. These moments of calm can make all the difference, turning the tide on pain and stress.

INCORPORATING GENTLE EXERCISE WITHOUT EXACERBATING PAIN

You are standing at the edge of your living room, contemplating whether today's the day you'll finally tackle that exercise routine you've been putting off. Chronic pain can make exercise daunting, but gentle exercise can be one of your greatest allies. It's like tending to a garden—small, regular efforts yield blooms of increased mobility and reduced discomfort over time. Picture this: moving through a series of low-impact exercises that don't leave you feeling like you've just run a marathon but instead leave you feeling a bit more alive and in tune with your body. These exercises decrease inflammation, a key player in the chronic pain orchestra, while boosting your mobility. It's a win-win,

Imagine starting your day with a brisk walk, not a sprint, but a comfortable pace that lets you soak in your surroundings. Walking is the unsung hero of exercise—a simple, low-impact activity that sets your joints in motion without overwhelming them. Swimming or water aerobics are equally fantastic, with the water acting as a gentle cushion, supporting your body and reducing stress on those aching joints. It's like floating on a cloud, where movements feel effortless and liberating. And for those days when the weather's not cooperating, or you just want a change of pace, consider cycling on a stationary bike. It's a great way to get your heart rate up while being kind to your body.

Strengthening exercises play a crucial role, too. Focusing on core muscles stabilizes your joints, making them less injury-prone. Think of your core as the trunk of a tree, providing the necessary support for all your branches—your limbs—to stretch and sway without snapping. Gentle Pilates or modified yoga routines can help build this strength, offering a structured yet flexible approach to enhance your stability. They're not about contorting into pretzel-like shapes but about mindful movements that build resilience and confidence.

Before diving into any exercise routine, it's wise to consult with a healthcare provider. Specific movements can aggravate certain conditions, and getting the green light ensures you're on the right track. Once you've got the go-ahead, remember that consistency is critical. Regular exercise routines, even brief, can dramatically improve your pain levels and overall health. It's about creating a habit that becomes a part of your lifestyle, not an occasional effort.

Incorporating gentle exercise into your daily routine isn't just about physical benefits; it's a mental boost, too. The endorphins released during these activities can help lift your mood, making pain more manageable and life a bit brighter. So lace up those sneakers, slip into your swimsuit, or unroll your yoga mat, and take that first step. With each movement, you're not just exercising; you're reclaiming a part of yourself that chronic pain tried to steal away. Moving is essential, but so is building a supportive healthcare team.

CHAPTER 9
BUILDING A SUPPORTIVE HEALTHCARE TEAM

Have you ever tried to assemble a piece of flat-pack furniture without the instructions, only to end up with screws left over and a wobbly table? Finding the right healthcare provider can feel like that, except we're discussing your health and well-being instead of a rickety table. Pain management isn't just a side gig for these folks; it's their main act. Having someone on your team who knows their way around the complex maze of chronic pain is crucial. You want someone who understands the intricacies of your condition and speaks your language, metaphorically and literally. This is where empathy and communication skills come into play. A provider who listens genuinely cares, and has a knack for explaining things in a way that doesn't require a medical degree is worth their weight in gold. Specialization in chronic pain is another feather in their cap, ensuring they can tailor treatments to your needs.

Finding such a provider might feel like searching for a needle in a haystack, but fear not! There are strategies to simplify the process. Start by checking credentials and certifications to ensure your provider has the necessary training and experience, especially with your type of pain. Patient reviews and testimonials can also be incredibly insightful. They're like the Yelp reviews of the medical world, offering a glimpse into other patients' experiences. Online directories and resources can be handy tools in your search, providing lists of specialists in your area. Don't hesitate to ask for recommendations from those in your circle who might have walked this path before you. Their insights could lead you to the healthcare provider who becomes your greatest ally.

In pain management, a multidisciplinary approach is often the secret sauce. Think of it as assembling an all-star team where each member brings their expertise. This team might include pain specialists, physiotherapists, and mental health professionals, among others, all collaborating to provide comprehensive care. Each specialist contributes a piece of the puzzle, addressing all aspects of your pain. This collaboration enhances treatment outcomes, creating a more holistic approach that considers pain's physical, psychological, and emotional facets. It's like having a pit crew in a race; each member focuses on a different aspect of your well-being, working together to keep you on track.

When preparing for initial consultations, a little homework goes a long way. Create a list of questions and concerns to discuss with your provider. This ensures you cover all your bases and keep all stones unturned. Bring relevant medical records and pain diaries to provide a comprehensive picture of your journey. These documents can give your provider valuable insights into your condition and help tailor a treatment plan that's just right for you. Setting clear expectations for treatment goals is also crucial. Discuss what you hope to achieve through this partnership and ensure your provider is on the same page. It's a collaborative effort, and open communication sets the stage for a successful relationship.

Interactive Element: Questions to Ask Your Healthcare Provider

Consider including these questions during your initial consultation to help guide the conversation:

- What experience do you have in treating my specific type of pain?
- How do you approach pain management?
- Are there any new treatments or therapies you would recommend?
- How can we monitor my progress together?
- What can I do between visits to manage my pain effectively?

BENEFITS OF A MULTIDISCIPLINARY HEALTHCARE TEAM

Imagine assembling a dream team, each member a superhero in their field, ready to tackle the villain that is chronic pain. That's what a multidisciplinary healthcare team offers—a collective of skilled professionals who bring their unique expertise to the table. Pain specialists, often the team captains, have the knowledge and experience to navigate the complexities of pain management. They coordinate care, ensuring each aspect of your treatment plan aligns with your needs. Their goal is not just to mask the pain but to address the root causes, seeking long-term relief and improved quality of life.

Physical therapists, the body's mechanics focus on movement and function. They help you strengthen muscles and improve mobility, teaching exercises to alleviate pain and prevent further injury. Think of them as the architects of your physical well-being, designing a regimen that supports your body's healing. They work closely with you to develop personalized plans that adapt as your needs change, empowering you to participate actively in your recovery. Their guidance can transform daily tasks from daunting obstacles into manageable activities.

Mental health professionals, the mind's navigators, play a crucial role in this ensemble. They provide strategies to cope with the emotional toll of chronic pain, offering tools to manage stress, anxiety, and depression. Addressing the psychological aspects of pain they help reduce its impact on your life. Their support provides a safe space to explore feelings and develop resilience. It's not just about surviving pain but finding ways to thrive despite it.

Together, this team forms a support network that addresses the multifaceted nature of chronic pain. They collaborate, communicate, and integrate their skills, ensuring you receive comprehensive care that considers your physical, emotional, and social needs. With their combined efforts, you're not battling pain alone; you have a dedicated team behind you, each member committed to helping you live your best life. This collaborative approach enhances treatment outcomes, turning the daunting journey of pain management into a path paved with understanding and hope.

JOINING COMMUNITIES: FINDING STRENGTH IN SHARED EXPERIENCES

Living with chronic pain can sometimes feel like you're navigating a labyrinth alone. But imagine turning a corner and finding others who understand exactly what you're going through. That's the magic of community support. Connecting with those who share similar experiences can be a lifeline, offering both emotional support and practical advice. It's like finding a club where everyone speaks your language. Shared knowledge becomes a powerful tool as you exchange tips and strategies that have worked for others. Emotional validation is equally invaluable. Knowing you're not alone in this battle can lift a weight off your shoulders and replace it with a sense of belonging.

You can explore various types of support communities, each offering its own flavor of camaraderie. Online forums and social media groups for chronic pain are like bustling virtual cafes where you can pop in anytime for a chat. They provide a space to ask questions, share experiences, and find solace in knowing you're not alone. Local support groups organized by healthcare facilities offer face-to-face interactions, allowing for deeper connections and immediate support. The U.S. Pain Foundation is another resource that connects you with a broader network, offering programs and events tailored to your needs.

Choosing the right community is crucial. It's like finding the right pair of shoes—comfort and fit matter. Evaluate community rules and member interactions to ensure the group aligns with your values. A positive and supportive environment is critical. You want a space where you feel safe to share and where negativity is checked at the door. When you find that fit, dive in; active participation and contribution can transform your experience. Share your personal stories and coping strategies, and don't hesitate to offer support and encouragement to fellow members. It's a two-way street; your involvement can make a difference for you and others walking the same path.

COMMUNITY SUPPORT GROUPS AND RESOURCES

Imagine a room filled with people who genuinely understand what you're going through. That's the magic of support groups. They offer a haven where shared experiences and empathy flow freely. When you're surrounded by others who get it, the feeling of isolation starts to melt away. It's like finding your tribe, people who speak the same language of pain and perseverance. These groups are more than just a place to vent; they're a treasure trove of coping strategies, offering new ways to manage pain you might not have considered. The reduction in loneliness is palpable as you realize you're not navigating this journey alone. Instead, you're part of a community that walks alongside you, sharing your victories and challenges.

Finding the right support group can take a bit of sleuthing. Online platforms like Facebook and Reddit are bustling hubs where you can connect with others from the comfort of your home. Local hospitals and community centers often host groups tailored to chronic pain, offering in-person connection. When evaluating options, consider the group dynamics and the credentials of facilitators. A supportive environment is critical, where respect and understanding are the order of the day. Finding a group that aligns with your values and where you feel comfortable sharing your experiences is essential.

Peer mentoring adds another layer of support, offering the chance to connect one-on-one with someone who's been in your shoes. It's like having a guide who can offer personalized advice and encouragement. Finding a mentor through support networks can provide insights tailored to your unique challenges. These relationships often result in profound, meaningful connections that go beyond the surface, offering a sense of camaraderie and shared resilience.

Beyond traditional support groups, community resources abound. Educational workshops and seminars can provide valuable insights into managing chronic pain, equipping you with new tools and perspectives. Public health services might offer additional support, from counseling to physical therapy. Community programs often include recreational activities designed for those with chronic pain, offering a chance to enjoy activities that bring joy without worrying about exacerbating symptoms.

Consider Lisa's story, a member who once felt isolated by her pain. Through her local support group, she found not only friendship but also practical strategies that transformed her approach to pain management. Her story is a testament to the power of community support, illustrating how shared experiences can lead to newfound strength and understanding. Nutrition and chronic pain will be discussed next in Chapter 10.

CHAPTER 10
NUTRITION AND CHRONIC PAIN

Picture your body as a bustling city, where each meal you consume is a building block. Some foods construct beautiful parks and efficient roads, easing traffic flow, while others erect unsightly traffic jams that cause endless honking and frustration. This analogy captures the essence of how your diet influences inflammation, a key player in chronic pain. Inflammation is your body's natural response to injury or stress. Still, when it becomes chronic, it can exacerbate pain, much like that never-ending construction work on the highway that never seems to finish. It's as if your body is stuck in a perpetual state of repair, sending out an army of inflammatory cells that, instead of fixing the problem, just create more chaos.

Certain foods have the uncanny ability to either fan the flames of inflammation or douse them with a soothing balm. Imagine your diet as a seesaw, with inflammatory foods on one side and anti-inflammatory foods on the other. Chronic pain can intensify when the balance tips towards inflammation, making it harder to manage. Foods high in saturated fats, refined sugars, and processed ingredients can act like gasoline on a fire, amplifying inflammation and discomfort. Conversely, a diet rich in anti-inflammatory foods can act like a gentle rain, cooling the flames and offering relief.

So, what are these magical anti-inflammatory foods that can help restore balance? Let's start with omega-3-rich foods, the super-heroes of the dietary world. Salmon, with its succulent, fatty goodness, and flaxseeds, tiny but mighty, are packed with omega-3 fatty acids. These nutrients are like peacekeepers, reducing inflammation and promoting heart health. Adding them to your meals can feel like giving your body a soothing hug from the inside. Leafy greens, such as spinach and kale, are another powerhouse. They're the unsung heroes of the vegetable aisle, brimming with vitamins and antioxidants that combat inflammation. Think of them as the green warriors that fight off the pesky inflammatory invaders.

Nuts and seeds, particularly almonds and walnuts, come into play as nature's portable snacks. They're rich in healthy fats and antioxidants, making them both delicious and beneficial. Picture them as tiny shields, protecting your body from the ravages of inflammation. And let's not forget berries, those sweet, juicy gems that add a burst of flavor to any dish. Blueberries and strawberries are packed with antioxidants, acting like tiny firefighters that quell the flames of pain. Incorporating these foods into your diet can be a game-changer, offering a natural way to combat inflammation.

Exploring anti-inflammatory diets can provide a structured approach to pain management. The Mediterranean diet, emphasizing whole foods, healthy fats, and lean proteins, is like a culinary vacation to a sun-drenched island, where every meal feels like a celebration. This diet has been shown to reduce inflammation and improve heart health, offering a holistic approach to wellness. Similarly, the DASH diet, which stands for Dietary Approaches to

Stop Hypertension, focuses on reducing sodium intake and increasing consumption of fruits, vegetables, and lean proteins. It's a practical plan that helps with blood pressure and reduces inflammation, making it a valuable ally in managing chronic pain.

Incorporating these anti-inflammatory foods into your daily meals doesn't have to be a chore. Imagine starting your day with a smoothie packed with spinach, flaxseeds, and a handful of berries, setting the tone for a vibrant, energetic day. Or consider a lunchtime salad with kale, salmon, and a sprinkle of walnuts drizzled with a tangy vinaigrette. These meals don't just nourish your body; they also delight your taste buds, making healthy eating an enjoyable experience.

Interactive Element: Recipe for Anti-Inflammatory Bliss

Try this simple, delicious recipe: Berry Nut Oatmeal Bowl. Cook a serving of oats and top with a mix of blueberries, strawberries, a tablespoon of flaxseeds, and a handful of almonds. Drizzle with a touch of honey or maple syrup for sweetness. This breakfast not only tastes heavenly but also kicks inflammation to the curb.

Regarding grocery shopping, think of your cart as your arsenal against pain. Focus on the store's perimeters, where fresh produce, lean proteins, and wholesome grains reside. Plan your meals in advance, prepping ingredients like chopped veggies and portioned nuts to make weekday meals a breeze. Maintaining consistency in dietary habits is like practicing a new skill—it gets easier and more rewarding with time. By embracing these nutritional changes, you can take a proactive step in managing chronic pain.

THE GUT-PAIN CONNECTION

Imagine your gut as a bustling metropolis, teeming with trillions of tiny inhabitants known as gut microbiota. These microscopic residents aren't just loitering around; they're busy maintaining harmony and order within your digestive system. The gut-brain axis is a fascinating two-way communication highway that connects this bustling metropolis with your brain. This connection is pivotal in modulating pain and mood, almost like a long-distance relationship where both parties influence each other's well-being. When your gut is healthy, it sends positive signals to your brain, which can help reduce pain perception and even lift your spirits. Conversely, if your gut is in disarray, it can exacerbate pain and lead to mood swings, making you feel like you're on an emotional roller coaster. This intricate dance between the gut and brain highlights the importance of gut health in managing chronic pain.

Fueling your gut with foods that promote a healthy environment is crucial to support this vital connection. Fermented foods such as yogurt and kimchi are like VIP guests at a party. They bring along probiotics, beneficial bacteria that support gut health and contribute to pain relief. Including them in your diet can feel like giving your gut a well-deserved spa day. Prebiotic-rich foods, including garlic and onions, act as the best friends of probiotics. They provide nourishment for these beneficial bacteria, ensuring they thrive and multiply. Think of prebiotics as the catering service at the gut's party, guaranteeing the probiotics are well-fed and happy. High-fiber foods like whole grains and legumes are the unsung heroes of gut health. They act as a cleaning crew, sweeping through the digestive tract, promoting regularity, and supporting a diverse microbiome. By incorporating these foods into your meals, you're not just feeding yourself; you're nurturing the tiny community within you that plays a crucial role in pain management.

Probiotics and prebiotics are like the dynamic duo of gut health supplements, each playing a unique yet complementary role. Probiotics introduce additional beneficial bacteria into your system, supporting gut balance and potentially reducing pain. They are the reinforcements, stepping in to bolster the gut's defenses. Incorporating probiotics through supplements or fermented foods can enhance gut health, promoting a stable environment that communicates positively with the brain. On the other hand, prebiotics are the support system for probiotics. They act as fuel, nourishing these beneficial bacteria and helping them thrive. Including prebiotics in your diet is like ensuring the probiotics have a constant supply of energy to keep the gut in tip-top shape.

Despite your best efforts to nourish your gut, certain foods can act like party crashers, disrupting the balance and potentially triggering pain. Processed sugars and refined carbs are notorious for causing gut havoc. They can lead to an overgrowth of harmful bacteria, tipping the scales toward inflammation and discomfort. Reducing their intake can be a game-changer, helping to restore gut harmony. Artificial sweeteners and additives, often found in processed foods, are like the uninvited guests who overstay their welcome. They can irritate the gut lining, leading to discomfort and pain. Opting for natural sweeteners or whole food alternatives can help keep these party crashers at bay. Gluten-containing grains, for some, can be a source of irritation. Substituting them with gluten-free options like quinoa or rice can alleviate gut distress, ensuring the digestive system remains happy and healthy.

By understanding the gut-pain connection, you empower yourself with the knowledge to make dietary choices that support your overall well-being. As you navigate this complex relationship, remember the importance of nurturing your gut microbiota with a diverse, balanced diet. In the next chapter, we will explore the role of technology and innovation in managing chronic pain, providing you with additional tools to enhance your journey toward relief.

CHAPTER 11
TECHNOLOGY AND CHRONIC PAIN

Imagine a world where your phone isn't just a device for scrolling through cat videos but a personal assistant helping you manage chronic pain. Welcome to the future of pain management, where technology is your ally. Mobile apps have taken the health world by storm, offering innovative solutions for tracking and managing chronic pain. These applications are like having a pocket therapist, doctor, and cheerleader all rolled into one. They empower you to track symptoms, remind you to take medication, and even integrate with your health records for a comprehensive view of your well-being. Apps like Curable and Bearable offer features such as guided exercises, pain logs, and trend analysis designed to help you better understand and manage your pain. With user testimonials singing praises of newfound control and clarity, it's clear that these digital tools are making a real difference in people's lives.

Wearable technology, on the other hand, literally brings the future to your wrist. Devices like smartwatches and fitness trackers provide real-time data that can be invaluable for managing chronic pain. Heart rate monitors, for example, are more than just a way to see how fast your heart races during a thriller movie. They can help you manage stress, a known exacerbator of pain. By keeping tabs on your heart rate, you can learn to recognize stress patterns and employ techniques to calm your body before pain spikes. Activity trackers are equally helpful, encouraging you to move just enough to keep your body limber without overdoing it. They act as your personal coach, nudging you to take those extra steps or reminding you to stretch after sitting too long. Sleep trackers, meanwhile, are like having a sleep detective on your wrist, helping you uncover patterns in your rest—or lack thereof—that might contribute to your pain.

Collecting data through these apps and wearables paints a detailed picture of your health landscape. It's like turning on the lights in a dim room, revealing insights that were once hidden. When shared with healthcare providers, this data becomes a powerful tool, allowing for tailored interventions to improve outcomes vastly. Patterns emerge, highlighting potential pain triggers or the effectiveness of specific treatments. It's like having a crystal ball, offering glimpses into what might come next and how to prepare. Identifying these patterns can lead to proactive strategies, reducing the frequency and intensity of pain episodes.

Choosing the right technology, however, can feel overwhelming with so many options available. It's like standing in the cereal aisle, facing a hundred boxes promising something special. To make the best choice, consider app usability and features matching your needs. You may prefer an app with a simple interface or one that offers robust data analysis. For wearables, think about functionalities that align with your lifestyle. Do you need constant reminders to move, or do you seek detailed sleep reports? Comparing popular wearables like the Apple Watch, Fitbit, or Garmin can help you decide which device will become your new daily companion.

Interactive Element: Technology Selection Checklist

- What are my primary goals for using an app or wearable? (e.g., tracking symptoms, managing stress)
- How important is the ease of use? (Consider your comfort level with technology)
- What features are essential for me? (e.g., heart rate monitoring, symptom tracking)
- What feedback have other users provided? (Look for reviews or testimonials)
- How does the technology integrate with other tools I use? (Consider compatibility with existing devices)

Armed with the right tools, you're managing pain and mastering it. Technology offers a new frontier where data and insights empower you to take control, turning chronic pain management into a personalized, proactive endeavor.

VIRTUAL REALITY AS A PAIN RELIEF TOOL

Imagine strapping on a headset and being transported to a serene beach, where the ocean waves gently lap at the shore, and the sun's warmth melts away your tension. This isn't just a fantasy—it's the reality offered by virtual reality (VR) technology. VR has emerged as a promising tool for managing chronic pain, leveraging its immersive experiences to alter pain perception. By engaging the senses and capturing the mind's focus, VR can distract from the persistent throb of pain, creating a mental barrier that makes discomfort less pronounced. It's like giving your brain a mini-vacation from the relentless awareness of pain. Programs designed specifically for chronic pain use this distraction technique to significant effect, offering experiences tailored to soothe and engage simultaneously. Whether a guided meditation in a tranquil forest or a playful exploration of an animated world, VR provides a refuge that can change how pain is experienced.

In clinical settings, VR's applications are expanding, with hospitals and rehabilitation centers integrating this technology into their pain management protocols. Case studies abound with stories of patients who have found relief through VR-assisted therapy, each narrative adding weight to the growing body of evidence supporting its use. Physiotherapy and occupational therapy have embraced VR as a complementary tool to enhance traditional rehabilitation exercises. Imagine performing physical therapy exercises not in a sterile room but within a vibrant virtual environment that makes the process engaging and less daunting. This integration can lead to improved patient compliance and outcomes, as the novelty and engagement of VR make therapy sessions something to look forward to rather than dread.

Research backs up these promising anecdotes with randomized controlled trials and longitudinal studies underscoring VR's efficacy in reducing pain. Studies show that VR can provide significant pain relief, with effects observed immediately or within a month of treatment. This isn't just a temporary fix; it's a tool that can rewire how pain is processed, potentially leading to longer-lasting benefits. The concept of cortical re-patterning comes into play here, where VR's immersive experiences might help the brain reorganize its response to pain, reducing its intensity. These findings are a beacon of hope for those who have long sought effective, non-pharmacological options for managing chronic pain.

However, as with any innovative solution, accessibility and cost considerations must be addressed. While increasingly available, VR technology can still pose financial barriers for some. High-end VR systems can be expensive, limiting access for individuals and healthcare facilities with limited budgets. Yet, the market is evolving, and more affordable home-use options are emerging. Some initiatives aim to increase access to VR technology in underserved areas, recognizing its potential for improving quality of life. These efforts are crucial for ensuring that VR's benefits aren't confined to those who can afford the latest gadgets but are available to anyone who might benefit from this transformative approach to pain management.

As we explore technology's role in chronic pain, it's clear that VR offers a unique blend of innovation and practicality, transforming how we perceive and manage discomfort. However, the journey doesn't end here. As we move forward, we'll continue to explore how these cutting-edge tools can fit into the broader landscape of chronic pain management, offering hope and relief to those who need it most. In the next chapter, we'll discuss the importance of exercise and mobility.

CHAPTER 12
EXERCISE AND MOBILITY

Imagine your body as an orchestra, with each muscle, joint, and bone playing its part to create a harmonious symphony of movement. Chronic pain, however, can be like that one rogue violinist playing off-key, throwing the whole ensemble off balance. But fear not! With the right exercises, we can help that violinist find its rhythm again, transforming discord into a melody of mobility. Let's explore how gentle exercises can ease the burden of chronic pain and restore harmony to your body.

Low-impact exercises are like the gentle lullaby of the exercise world, offering a way to stay active without sending your joints into a tizzy. Take swimming, for instance. It's like a full-body hug from the water, supporting your weight while letting you glide effortlessly. Swimming and aquatic therapy provide resistance that strengthens muscles without straining them, making it an excellent choice for those with joint pain. Walking on even surfaces is another option; taking your joints on a leisurely stroll through a park ensures they don't encounter any unexpected bumps. It's gentle, consistent, and a fantastic way to keep your body moving.

Then there's cycling on stationary bikes, which offers the thrill of a ride without the risk of outdoor obstacles. It's a low-impact workout that strengthens your legs and improves cardiovascular health, all from the comfort of your home or gym.

Stretching is the unsung hero of exercise routines, often overlooked but oh-so-essential. It's like giving your muscles a good morning stretch, preparing them for the day ahead. Regular stretching routines can enhance flexibility and reduce stiffness, making movement more comfortable. Dynamic stretching, which involves moving while stretching, is excellent for warming up the body. It's like gently waking up your muscles, saying, "Hey, it's time to get moving!" Static stretching, however, involves holding a stretch for a period, allowing muscles to lengthen and relax. Think of it as a soothing sigh of relief for your muscles after a long day. Targeted stretches for common pain areas such as the lower back or shoulders can be particularly beneficial, helping address specific discomforts. Morning and evening stretching routines can bookend your day with relaxation and readiness, setting a positive tone for your body.

If you want to add mindfulness to your exercise, Tai Chi and Qigong are your go-to practices. These ancient Chinese exercises combine slow, deliberate movements with controlled breathing, offering a unique blend of physical and mental benefits. Tai Chi is like a gentle dance, with each movement flowing into the next, promoting balance and coordination. It's particularly beneficial for chronic pain sufferers, as it eases joint tension and strengthens muscles. Breathing techniques complement the movements, creating a meditative state that reduces stress and anxiety. Classes tailored for beginners and those with limited mobility ensure that everyone can join the dance, making it accessible to all.

Before you dive into these exercises, let's talk about safety. Proper warm-up and cool-down routines are crucial, acting like a safety net for your muscles and joints. Warm-ups gradually increase your heart rate and blood flow, preparing your body for exercise. Conversely, cool-downs help your body return to its resting state, reducing the risk of injury. Monitoring your pain levels during exercise is essential to avoid overexertion. Your body will let you know when enough is enough, so listen to it. Supportive footwear and equipment can make a difference, providing the stability and comfort needed for a safe workout.

Reflection Section: Crafting Your Exercise Plan

Take a moment to reflect on the exercises that resonate with you. Consider your current abilities, interests, and goals. Write down a plan that includes your preferred exercises, stretching routines, and any safety measures you'll take. This plan can serve as a roadmap, guiding you toward improved mobility and reduced pain.

Exercise doesn't have to be a chore; it can be a joyful part of your day that empowers you to take control of your pain. By incorporating these gentle exercises into your routine, you're not just moving your body—you're moving toward a life where pain takes a backseat to strength and resilience.

THE IMPORTANCE OF PACING AND REST

In chronic pain, pacing is your trusty sidekick, the wise guide that helps you navigate the tumultuous terrain of daily life. Think of pacing as a dance—a delicate balance between activity and rest. It's not about sprinting to the finish line but finding a rhythm that allows you to move forward without stumbling. Setting realistic activity goals is the first step in this dance. Break tasks into manageable segments instead of tackling everything at once, much like savoring a meal one bite at a time. This approach prevents you from overextending yourself and keeps fatigue at bay. Listening to your body's signals is crucial; it's like having an internal GPS that warns you when it's time to pause. Ignoring these signals can increase pain and exhaustion, turning even the simplest tasks into huge efforts.

Rest isn't just a passive activity; it's an integral part of managing chronic pain. Just as a car needs fuel, your body needs rest to recharge and function optimally. Scheduled rest breaks throughout the day act as pit stops, allowing you to refuel and continue your journey with renewed energy. These breaks don't have to be lengthy; even a few minutes can make a difference. Stimulating activities such as meditation or reading can enhance these rest periods, providing a mental escape and reducing stress. Imagine creating a restful environment—a sanctuary where your mind and body can unwind. Whether it's a cozy corner with soft lighting or a quiet room free from distractions, this space becomes a haven for recovery. A restful environment sets the stage for optimal healing, allowing you to emerge rejuvenated and ready to face the world.

Enter the "Spoon Theory," a clever metaphor that captures the essence of energy conservation for those living with chronic pain. Imagine starting each day with a limited number of spoons, each representing a unit of energy. Every task, from brushing your teeth to running errands, costs a spoon or two. Even small tasks might require more spoons on high-pain days, forcing you to ration your energy carefully. Allocating spoons for daily tasks becomes a prioritization exercise, ensuring you have enough power for the essentials. It's about making conscious choices, deciding what truly matters, and letting go of what doesn't. This approach empowers you to take control of your energy and avoid the dreaded crash that comes from overexertion.

Let me share a story about Alex, a fellow chronic pain warrior who discovered the power of pacing. Alex starts each day with a plan, allocating spoons for tasks like work, exercise, and family time. By breaking tasks into smaller chunks, Alex avoids the temptation to push through pain, instead taking breaks to rest and recharge. A typical day might involve a morning walk, followed by a short break for meditation. In the afternoon, Alex tackles work projects in focused bursts, interspersed with restful activities like reading or listening to music. By the end of the day, Alex had accomplished more with less pain, thanks to the strategic use of spoons.

Another inspiring story is that of Maria, who transformed her quality of life through energy management. Once overwhelmed by her job and family demands, Maria learned to listen to her body's cues. She set realistic goals and embraced the concept of pacing, allowing herself to rest without guilt. Maria's newfound approach enabled her to participate in activities she once thought impossible, like attending social events or taking short trips. Her story reminds us that pacing isn't about doing less; it's about doing more of what matters with the energy you have.

These stories illustrate the transformative potential of pacing and rest in managing chronic pain. By embracing these strategies, you can enhance your quality of life, reduce pain, and reclaim activities that bring joy and fulfillment. Remember, pacing isn't a sign of weakness; it's a testament to your strength and resilience, a way to honor your body's needs while living life to the fullest. Mindfulness and meditation can also be valuable tools in managing chronic pain.

CHAPTER 13
MINDFULNESS AND MEDITATION

Picture yourself standing in front of a grand, ancient library, its shelves filled with the wisdom of ages. This library is your mind, and mindfulness is the key that unlocks its doors. Mindfulness, as defined by Jon Kabat-Zinn, is "awareness that arises through paying attention, on purpose, in the present moment, non-judgmentally." It's about living in the now, not in the past of regrets or future of worries. For those of us managing chronic pain, mindfulness offers a sanctuary of peace, a way to step back from pain and observe it without letting it consume us. It's not about ignoring pain but understanding it as part of your life's tapestry. This approach can reduce stress and enhance emotional regulation, turning what once felt like an unmanageable storm into a series of gentle waves.

Developing mindful awareness doesn't require you to become a monk. Instead, it involves integrating simple practices into your daily routine. Imagine turning your meals into a sensory experience—this is mindful eating. Instead of scarfing down food while staring at a screen, you savor each bite, noticing flavors, textures, and aromas. It's like giving your taste buds a front-row seat to a culinary concert, enhancing your eating experience and awareness. Then there's mindful walking, where each step becomes a dance with the earth, grounding you and connecting you to the world. You might feel the breeze on your skin or hear the crunch of leaves underfoot, leaving stress behind with each step. Mindful breathing, on the other hand, is your anchor in turbulent waters. Focusing on each inhale and exhale gives you a calming rhythm, a reminder that your breath remains steady and constant amidst the chaos.

Mindfulness-Based Stress Reduction (MBSR) is like the master mindfulness class, offering structured support for chronic pain sufferers. An MBSR course typically spans eight weeks, offering a blend of meditation, gentle yoga, and group discussions. It's like attending a fitness boot camp for your mind, where you train to respond to pain with acceptance rather than resistance. Research supports MBSR's effectiveness, with studies showing significant improvements in pain reduction and quality of life for participants, especially those grappling with chronic headaches. By focusing on the present, MBSR helps you develop coping strategies to make a difference.

Incorporating mindfulness into your daily life doesn't have to be a daunting task. Start small by setting reminders for mindfulness breaks throughout your day. These can be as simple as pausing to take a few deep breaths or tuning into your surroundings for a moment. Creating a mindfulness corner at home can also be incredibly helpful—a cozy nook where you can retreat for regular practice. Maybe it's a chair by the window or a mat on the floor, whatever makes you feel calm and centered. Mindfulness apps can also support your practice, offering guided sessions and exercises tailored to your needs. They're like having a mindfulness coach in your pocket, ready to guide you whenever you need a moment of peace.

Interactive Element: Mindful Moment Checklist

Consider creating a checklist to remind yourself of mindful practices you can incorporate into your day:

- Take three mindful breaths before getting out of bed.
- Savor your morning beverage, noticing its warmth and aroma.
- Practice mindful walking during a break, focusing on your steps.
- Set aside five minutes to sit quietly and breathe deeply.
- Reflect on one thing you're grateful for before bedtime.

By integrating these practices into your routine, you create a space where mindfulness can flourish, offering solace and strength amidst the challenges of chronic pain.

GUIDED MEDITATION FOR PAIN MANAGEMENT

Imagine a world where you can transform the perception of pain into something more manageable. This is where guided meditation offers a fresh outlook on the sensations that often dominate your day. At its core, meditation works by influencing the brain and nervous system, acting like a gentle conductor guiding an orchestra. It helps your body switch from the 'fight or flight' mode to a more relaxed state. Brain scans have shown that meditation can decrease activity in areas linked to pain perception, allowing you to experience relief like turning down the volume on a blaring radio. Over time, meditation can enhance pain tolerance and build emotional resilience, helping you face challenges with renewed strength and optimism.

To begin your meditation practice, consider starting with a simple body scan. This technique invites you to focus on different parts of your body, starting from your toes and gradually working your way up. You might notice sensations of warmth, tingling, or even discomfort, but rather than judging them, you simply observe. It's like taking a mental inventory, acknowledging what's there without trying to change it. This heightened awareness promotes relaxation and can help release tension. Another approach is loving-kindness meditation, where you cultivate feelings of compassion and warmth towards yourself. You might silently repeat phrases like, "May I be safe, may I be happy, may I be free from pain." It's a gentle reminder that you deserve kindness, especially from yourself. Visualization techniques also offer comfort, allowing you to create mental imagery of a serene place, such as a peaceful beach or a tranquil forest, providing an escape from physical discomfort.

Consistency is critical to reaping the long-term benefits of meditation. Setting a regular schedule, even if it's just a few minutes a day, helps build discipline and integrate meditation into your routine. You might find it helpful to keep a meditation journal, noting your experiences, challenges, and any progress you observe. This practice tracks your journey and offers insights into patterns that might emerge. Perhaps you notice that your mind is restless on certain days or that you're more at ease after a session. These observations can guide your practice, helping you refine and adapt your approach.

In today's digital age, accessing guided meditations is easier than ever. Numerous online platforms offer free tracks tailored to chronic pain, providing guidance and support at your fingertips. Apps like Headspace or Calm allow you to customize sessions based on your preferences, offering everything from quick meditations to longer, immersive experiences. Community meditation groups or classes can also provide a shared space to practice, fostering a sense of connection and shared purpose.

Shifting gears, let's explore how Cognitive Behavioral Therapy (CBT) complements meditation in managing pain. CBT operates on the principle that our thoughts, feelings, and behaviors are interconnected. Changing thought patterns and behaviors can alter how we experience pain. One technique is cognitive restructuring, which involves identifying and challenging negative thoughts that amplify pain. For instance, the thought "I can't handle this pain" can be reframed to "This pain is challenging, but I have strategies to manage it." This shift reduces the emotional weight of pain, making it more bearable. Activity pacing, another CBT strategy, emphasizes balancing rest and activity, preventing flare-ups, and maintaining engagement in meaningful activities.

Research has consistently shown the efficacy of CBT in altering pain perception and improving mental health. Studies highlight its ability to reduce pain intensity and distress while also decreasing anxiety and depression. This dual impact makes CBT a powerful tool in the pain management arsenal. Accessing CBT resources has never been more convenient, with online programs offering structured guidance and flexibility. Finding a qualified therapist can also provide personalized support, tailoring strategies to fit your unique needs and circumstances.

By integrating meditation and CBT into your pain management plan, you cultivate a comprehensive approach that addresses both the mind and body. With these tools, you're managing pain and transforming your relationship with it. As we move forward, let's explore how these practices connect to the broader landscape of holistic pain management, offering hope and empowerment. As discussed in the next chapter, biofeedback can also help satisfy that need.

CHAPTER 14

BIOFEEDBACK AND CHRONIC PAIN

Imagine if your body came with its own dashboard, much like a car. Instead of oil and engine lights, you'd have stress, muscle tension, and heart rate indicators. Biofeedback is like that dashboard, offering a window into your body's inner workings that you never knew you needed. It's a non-invasive therapy that uses monitoring devices to help you become aware of physiological processes, those behind-the-scenes activities happening inside you without your conscious input. By providing real-time feedback, biofeedback empowers you to take the wheel, helping you learn to control these processes. This isn't about Jedi mind tricks or magical cures; it's about harnessing the power of data to guide you toward relaxation and pain relief.

Biofeedback measures physiological functions such as heart rate, muscle tension, and skin temperature. Think of it as a mirror reflecting your body's responses to stress and pain. As you watch these metrics change, you recognize patterns and learn how your body reacts to different situations. This awareness is the first step toward self-regulation. By seeing how your heart rate spikes during stress or how your skin temperature drops when you're anxious, you can practice techniques to bring these metrics back to baseline. It's like having a personal trainer for your autonomic nervous system, encouraging you to flex those relaxation muscles.

Various biofeedback devices cater to different needs, each offering a unique perspective on your physiological state. Electromyography (EMG) focuses on muscle tension, using sensors to track your muscles' tightness or relaxedness. It's beneficial for chronic back pain or tension headaches, where muscle tension plays a significant role. Thermal biofeedback monitors skin temperature, providing insights into stress responses and blood flow. As stress tends to constrict blood vessels, causing lower skin temperatures, learning to raise your skin temperature can be a cue for relaxation. Galvanic skin response sensors measure sweat gland activity, highlighting how your body reacts to stress at a more granular level. Heart rate variability monitors are stress detectives, assessing how your heart rate changes with breathing patterns, offering a direct link to your stress and relaxation cycles.

The benefits of biofeedback in managing chronic pain are like finding that extra gear you didn't know your bicycle had. It offers a way to reduce muscle tension and the associated pain, providing a direct avenue for relief. By enhancing relaxation responses, biofeedback helps you tap into your body's natural calming mechanisms, akin to finding the 'off' switch for stress. It improves stress management skills, teaching you how to respond rather than react, turning mountains back into molehills. With increased awareness of pain triggers and patterns, you become your own detective, able to identify and address the root causes of discomfort rather than just the symptoms.

Evidence supporting biofeedback's efficacy is both robust and promising. Clinical trials have demonstrated significant reductions in the frequency and intensity of migraines, offering hope to those who have tried everything else without success. For people living with fibromyalgia, biofeedback shows promise, particularly in reducing pain intensity, and the journey doesn't stop there. Longitudinal studies tracking biofeedback's impact on chronic pain management reveal sustained improvements, proving that this isn't just a flash-in-the-pan solution but a viable long-term strategy. The meta-analysis of studies highlights a consistent reduction in pain intensity and associated symptoms, making a solid case for biofeedback as a cornerstone in managing chronic pain.

Interactive Element: Biofeedback Device Cheat Sheet

Here's a quick reference to help you understand which biofeedback device might suit your needs:

- EMG Biofeedback: Best for muscle tension issues, such as tension headaches or chronic neck pain.
- Thermal Biofeedback: Ideal for stress-related conditions, as it focuses on skin temperature and blood flow.
- Galvanic Skin Response Sensors: Great for anxiety management, providing insights into sweat gland activity.
- Heart Rate Variability Monitors: Perfect for overall stress and relaxation tracking, linking heart rate to breathing patterns.

With this cheat sheet in hand, you're better equipped to explore biofeedback's possibilities. Step into this world of self-discovery and control, and find the balance between mind, body, and pain.

IMPLEMENTING BIOFEEDBACK TECHNIQUES

Choosing the proper biofeedback method is akin to picking the perfect pair of shoes. It has to fit your needs, feel comfortable, and be something you'll use regularly. Start by considering your specific pain symptoms. An EMG device might be your go-to for muscle tension headaches, while those dealing with stress-induced temperature changes might benefit from thermal biofeedback. Accessibility is another crucial factor. Home devices offer convenience, but ensure they meet your technical comfort level. If you're not a tech fan, a more straightforward device might be more user-friendly. Consulting with a healthcare professional can provide personalized recommendations, ensuring you select a method that aligns with your health goals. These professionals can help interpret data and offer insights into your physiological responses, guiding you toward the most effective techniques.

Integrating biofeedback into your daily routine doesn't have to be a daunting task. Set up your biofeedback equipment in a quiet, comfortable space with minimal distractions. Begin by familiarizing yourself with the device—read manuals, watch tutorials, and learn how it functions. Once you're relaxed, start by measuring your baseline metrics. This initial data serves as a reference point, helping you to identify stress responses and track progress over time. As you interpret this feedback data, look for patterns. Do certain activities spike your heart rate or increase muscle tension? Use these insights to tailor your relaxation exercises. Guided by biofeedback readings, practice deep breathing, progressive muscle relaxation, or visualization techniques, adjusting as needed based on your physiological responses. Over time, these practices can become second nature, seamlessly woven into your life.

Professional biofeedback sessions can be a game-changer, offering depth and expertise that complements home practices. Working with a certified biofeedback practitioner provides a structured environment where you can explore advanced techniques under expert guidance. These sessions often begin with a comprehensive assessment, where the practitioner evaluates your specific needs and tailors the approach accordingly. With their help, you can achieve deeper states of relaxation, learning to control involuntary responses with greater precision. Professional sessions can also introduce more complex equipment or techniques that aren't feasible at home, broadening your toolkit and enhancing your self-regulation skills. The supportive environment of professional therapy provides accountability, ensuring you maintain momentum and stay committed to your biofeedback practice.

Success stories from those who have embraced biofeedback offer inspiration and proof of its potential. Take Jane, for instance, who suffered from debilitating tension headaches. She learned to identify tension patterns and implement relaxation techniques through regular biofeedback sessions, reducing her headache frequency and intensity. Or consider Mark, who battled anxiety and insomnia. By practicing heart rate variability biofeedback, he gained control over his stress responses, improving sleep quality and reducing anxiety levels. These narratives highlight the transformative power of biofeedback, illustrating how it can redefine the experience of chronic pain and stress. They serve as reminders that change is possible, even when pain feels insurmountable.

Consistency and patience are crucial to unlocking the full benefits of biofeedback. Like learning to play an instrument or mastering a new skill, progress takes time and dedication. Set realistic expectations and understand that biofeedback is not an overnight solution. It's a gradual process that requires regular practice and reflection. Track your changes diligently, noting improvements in pain levels, stress responses, and overall well-being. Celebrate small victories along the way, whether it's a day with less pain or a moment of calm amidst chaos. Recognize that each step forward is a testament to your commitment and resilience. By staying the course and honing your skills, you'll find that biofeedback becomes a powerful ally in your journey toward better health and greater control over your body and mind.

As we wrap up our exploration of biofeedback, remember that this technique offers a unique blend of insight, control, and empowerment. Understanding and influencing your physiological responses can make meaningful strides toward managing chronic pain. Biofeedback is not just about measuring; it's about learning and growing, equipping you with the tools to navigate life's challenges confidently and calmly. As we transition to the next chapter, we'll continue to explore how technology and innovation can further support and enhance your journey toward wellness. Common misconceptions about chronic pain will be discussed in Chapter 15.

CHAPTER 15
ADDRESSING COMMON MISCONCEPTIONS

Picture this: You're at a party, and someone starts talking about chronic pain. They look at you and say, "Isn't it all just in your head?" You resist the urge to roll your eyes and calmly sip your drink. This is just one of the many myths surrounding chronic pain—myths that can make living with it even more challenging. Let's debunk these misconceptions together, starting with the idea that chronic pain is merely psychological. It's not just a trick of the mind. Chronic pain is as real as you and me, with physical and neurological underpinnings that science has thoroughly documented.

The notion that chronic pain is all in your head is a stubborn myth that dismisses the authentic experiences of those who live with it. Conditions like fibromyalgia, for instance, present with invisible symptoms such as widespread pain and fatigue, making it easy for outsiders to overlook them. Yet, these conditions have a firm basis in the body's complex systems. Neurological pathways misfire and pain signals persist long after any initial injury has healed. The brain, in response, becomes a stage for this relentless drama, with neurons misbehaving like unruly teenagers. Scientific evidence supports the physiological nature of these conditions, demonstrating that chronic pain is a multifaceted phenomenon deeply entwined with our body's physical landscape.

Next, let's tackle the misconception that experiencing pain equates to weakness. Society often valorizes stoicism, but dealing with chronic pain is not a testament to one's frailty—quite the opposite. Chronic pain warriors are some of the strongest individuals you'll encounter, enduring daily battles with grit and determination. These individuals navigate life with a resilience that would put most to shame, adapting to challenges with resourcefulness. Societal attitudes, however, can sometimes equate visible strength with the ability to "push through," overlooking the quiet strength it takes to manage chronic pain. It's crucial to shift this narrative, recognizing that strength comes in many forms and that those living with chronic pain are anything but weak. Their daily perseverance and courage exemplify a strength that deserves admiration, not pity.

Another misconception worth addressing is the idea of a one-size-fits-all treatment for chronic pain. Imagine trying to fit into a pair of shoes two sizes too small. It doesn't work, and it certainly doesn't feel good. Chronic pain management is similar—it requires a personalized approach. What works wonders for one person might fall flat for another. Take, for example, two individuals with similar back pain symptoms. One might find relief through physical therapy and yoga, while the other might need a combination of medication and acupuncture. This individualized nature of treatment plans allows for effective management, as each person's pain story is unique. Emphasizing the need for personalized care underscores the importance of patient-centered approaches, where treatments are tailored to meet each individual's specific needs and circumstances.

Finally, there's the persistent belief that chronic pain must be visible to be legitimate. This is one of those myths that can make you want to shake your head in disbelief. Chronic pain is often invisible, lurking beneath the surface without apparent signs. Invisible illnesses, such as fibromyalgia or CRPS, challenge the notion that "seeing is believing," as they don't always show outward symptoms. Yet, the impact on daily life is significant, affecting everything from mobility to mental health. It's vital to believe patients when they describe their pain experiences, even if you can't see the evidence. Trusting their narratives and validating their feelings can make a world of difference, fostering empathy and understanding in a world that often demands proof. Chronic pain may be invisible, but its effects are undeniably authentic and deserving of compassion and attention.

BUILDING AWARENESS AND UNDERSTANDING

Chronic pain is not a monolith; it's a vast spectrum of conditions, each with its quirks and challenges. Some are well-known, like arthritis or migraines, while others lurk in the shadows, less understood and often misdiagnosed. Take, for example, Ehlers-Danlos syndrome, a connective tissue disorder that can cause joint pain and hypermobility, or trigeminal neuralgia, usually called a "suicide disease" due to the intense facial pain it causes. Then, there's interstitial cystitis, a condition that leads to chronic bladder pain. Imagine living with a condition where even the most basic bodily functions become painful. These disorders remind us that chronic pain isn't a one-size-fits-all issue. Each condition brings its hurdles, and those living with them often navigate a landscape of uncertainty and frustration. It's crucial to recognize this diversity, as understanding the vast array of chronic pain conditions allows us to support better those who face them daily.

Consider individuals like Tom, who battles the constant pain of cluster headaches, often described as more excruciating than childbirth, or Sarah, who deals with the unrelenting discomfort of fibromyalgia. This condition can make even a warm hug feel like a bear trap. Each story reveals a different aspect of the chronic pain spectrum, highlighting people's varied experiences and challenges. Tom's headaches come in cycles, wreaking havoc on his life, yet he pushes through with the help of specialized treatments and support from his family. Sarah, on the other hand, has learned to manage her fibromyalgia through a blend of medication, lifestyle changes, and a deep commitment to self-care. Their experiences remind us of the resilience and adaptability required to live with chronic pain, as well as the need for personalized treatment plans that cater to individual needs.

Fostering empathy and support for those living with chronic pain requires more than just understanding; it requires active listening and validation. When someone shares their pain story, the best thing you can offer is your ear and an open heart. Validate their experiences by acknowledging their feelings and avoiding the urge to offer unsolicited advice. Sometimes, saying, "I hear you, and I'm here for you," can mean the world. Practical support can also make a significant difference. Offer to help with daily tasks, run errands, or simply spend time together in ways that are comfortable for them. But remember, respect their boundaries. Overstepping with well-meaning advice or actions can be counterproductive, so always ask before you act.

Education plays a pivotal role in shifting societal perceptions of chronic pain. Initiatives and programs that promote awareness can change the narrative, fostering understanding and compassion. Organizations like the National Pain Advocacy Center are at the forefront, working tirelessly to educate the public and influence policy. Whether through community workshops, school programs, or online resources, educational outreach has successfully increased understanding. Take, for example, the impact of awareness campaigns that highlight the realities of living with chronic pain. These efforts have led to increased funding for research, better access to treatment, and a shift in how society views pain sufferers. By expanding our collective knowledge, we can create a more inclusive and supportive environment for those living with chronic pain.

Empowerment comes from knowledge and action, and you have the power to advocate for change. Get involved in advocacy groups and campaigns to improve chronic pain treatment options and policies. If you feel comfortable, share your personal story to raise awareness and drive policy change. Your voice can make a difference, offering insight and understanding to those unfamiliar with the struggles of chronic pain. Engaging in social media advocacy is also a powerful tool. Platforms like Twitter and Facebook provide opportunities to connect with others, share information, and amplify the conversation around chronic pain. Participating in these efforts, you help create a world where chronic pain is better understood and more effectively addressed.

As we wrap up this chapter, it's clear that awareness and understanding are crucial in reshaping the narrative around chronic pain. We can build a more compassionate society by acknowledging the diverse spectrum of conditions, fostering empathy, and promoting education. As we transition into the next chapter, we'll explore practical strategies for managing chronic pain with sleep strategies.

CHAPTER 16
SLEEP STRATEGIES FOR THOSE WITH CHRONIC PAIN

Imagine your bed as a luxurious five-star hotel suite with fluffy pillows and the world's most comfortable mattress. Yet, despite this ideal setup, you find yourself tossing and turning, unable to enjoy the restorative sleep your body desperately craves. Chronic pain has a way of turning even the coziest bed into a battlefield, where each movement feels like a skirmish, and sleep becomes an elusive dream. This chapter delves into the complex relationship between sleep and chronic pain, exploring how they intertwine in a dance that can soothe or exacerbate your discomfort.

THE CONNECTION BETWEEN SLEEP AND CHRONIC PAIN

The relationship between sleep and chronic pain is like a tango—intimately connected and often unpredictable. When sleep deprivation enters the picture, it amps up pain sensitivity, making even the gentlest touch feel like an assault. Think of it as having a broken volume knob on a stereo that only goes up, never down.

The less sleep you get, the higher the volume of your pain seems to be. According to research, insufficient sleep can disrupt various systems in your body, including the opioid system, which is crucial for moderating pain. This disruption diminishes your body's ability to inhibit pain, leaving you more vulnerable to its effects.

But there's more to this story. The monoaminergic system, involving neurotransmitters like serotonin and norepinephrine, also goes haywire with sleep deprivation. This system plays a significant role in both mood and pain regulation. When it's thrown off balance, you might be more sensitive to pain and irritable and anxious—like a bear woken up too early from hibernation. Dopamine, another key player, is essential for regulating both sleep and pain. Sleep deprivation may decrease dopaminergic activity, further increasing pain sensitivity and leaving you in a foggy, cranky state. It's like navigating a maze with a blindfold on —frustrating and exhausting.

Conversely, restorative sleep is your body's natural healer, working behind the scenes to repair the daily wear and tear. When you sleep well, your body releases growth hormones that aid in tissue repair and regeneration, helping you recover from the physical demands of the day. Restorative sleep also supports your immune system, making it more efficient at fighting inflammation, which is often a key contributor to chronic pain. It's like having a team of tiny repair workers who come in at night to fix everything that's gone awry during the day. Without adequate sleep, this repair process is compromised, leaving you more susceptible to the aches and pains that chronic pain brings.

In addition to these physiological benefits, restorative sleep profoundly impacts your cognitive and emotional well-being. It helps regulate mood, improve focus, and boost overall well-being. When well-rested, you're better equipped to handle stressors and challenges, including those pesky pain flare-ups that seem to come out of nowhere. It's as if sleep provides you with a suit of armor, allowing you to face the day with resilience and grace.

The interplay between sleep and chronic pain is further complicated by the body's stress-response system, known as the hypothalamus-pituitary-adrenal (HPA) axis. Sleep deficiency can disrupt this system, leading to increased levels of stress hormones like cortisol. Elevated cortisol levels can heighten pain perception and exacerbate feelings of anxiety and depression, creating a vicious cycle where pain and poor sleep feed off each other. Breaking this cycle requires a concerted effort to prioritize sleep and address the underlying factors that disrupt it.

Reflection Section: Sleep Journal

Consider starting a sleep journal to track your sleep patterns, noting any factors that may impact your rest, such as stress levels, caffeine intake, or pain episodes. Over time, this journal can help you identify trends and tailor your sleep strategies to suit your needs better, allowing you to reclaim your nights and wake up feeling refreshed and ready to tackle the day.

Understanding the intricate connection between sleep and chronic pain is the first step towards reclaiming your nights and improving your quality of life. By prioritizing restorative sleep, you can help your body heal and empower yourself to face each day with renewed energy and strength.

DISCUSSING COMMON SLEEP DISRUPTORS AND HOW TO MANAGE THEM

Let's talk about sleep, or rather, the lack of it, and the culprits behind those restless nights. Imagine your brain as a bustling city where caffeine is that unruly driver who won't stop honking. It keeps everything awake and buzzing long after rush hour is over. Caffeine, found in coffee, tea, energy drinks, and even chocolate, is a stimulant that blocks adenosine, a chemical that promotes sleep. That late-afternoon coffee might seem harmless, but studies show it can reduce your total sleep time by over an hour. The trick here is timing. Cutting off caffeine six hours before bedtime can make a world of difference. If you're looking for a pick-me-up in the afternoon, consider alternatives like herbal teas or a brisk walk to invigorate your senses without disrupting your sleep.

Now, let's address another sleep thief: electronic devices. These glowing screens are like your brain's version of a rave party, complete with strobe lights that disrupt your natural sleep rhythm. Blue light emitted by phones, tablets, and computers interferes with melatonin production, the hormone responsible for regulating sleep. It's like having a constant sunrise in your face when you should be winding down. To combat this, try implementing a digital curfew. Aim to turn off screens at least an hour before bed, giving your brain time to transition from the digital world to dreamland. If you must use devices, consider blue-light filters or night mode settings that reduce the impact on your sleep cycle. Swap that late-night screen time with calming activities like reading a book or listening to soothing music, creating a more serene path to slumber.

Stress and anxiety are the uninvited guests at the sleepover, whispering worry into your ear just as you're about to drift off. They have a knack for amplifying pain and making your mind race with thoughts of unfinished tasks and what-ifs. This is where journaling comes into play. Think of it as a brain dump to clear your mind of clutter before bed. Spend a few minutes jotting down your thoughts, concerns, and even moments of gratitude. This practice can help you process emotions and set aside worries until morning, like putting your brain on airplane mode for the night. It can also be a tool for reflection, helping you identify patterns or triggers affecting your sleep.

Meditation is another powerful ally in the quest for restful sleep. Picture it as a mental spa day, where your mind can unwind and recharge. Techniques like mindfulness and guided or body scan meditation can help you relax, reduce insomnia, and enhance inner peace. By focusing on your breath or visualizing tranquil scenes, you create a buffer against stress, allowing your mind to settle into a calm state. Regular practice can improve mood, relieve stress, and reduce anxiety—factors that often contribute to sleep disturbances. Meditation can be done at any time of day, but incorporating it into your bedtime routine can signal to your body that it's time to wind down.

These strategies, when combined, create a supportive framework for better sleep. Adjusting your caffeine habits, reducing screen time, and adopting practices like journaling and meditation can transform your nights from restless to restful. Small changes can lead to significant improvements, helping you reclaim the rest you need and deserve. Remember, sleep is not just a passive state but an active recovery and rejuvenation process.

As we wrap up this chapter, consider how these strategies might fit into your life. Sleep, like a well-tuned instrument, requires attention and care. Making minor tweaks to your routine can enhance your sleep quality, manage your pain more effectively, and improve your overall well-being. With these tools in your arsenal, you're better prepared to face the challenges of chronic pain with a clearer mind and a rested body. Speaking of challenges, the next chapter will delve into empowering the chronic pain warrior.

CHAPTER 17
EMPOWERING THE CHRONIC PAIN WARRIOR

You know, life with chronic pain can sometimes feel like a never-ending boxing match. Just when you think you've got it under control, it throws another punch. But within this relentless battle, some stories shine like beacons, offering hope and showing what's possible when resilience takes the lead. Let's dive into these tales of courage, starting with a veteran who found a new purpose through community support. After leaving the military, he faced the daunting task of rebuilding his life while wrestling with chronic pain. It was through a local veterans' group that he discovered the strength of shared experiences. These meetings weren't just about swapping stories; they were about building a network of support that helped him reclaim his life. Community support became his lifeline, offering both practical advice and emotional solidarity.

Then there's the single parent who, every day, juggles family responsibilities with a body that doesn't always cooperate. Picture this: school runs, dinner prep, and bedtime stories, all while managing pain that refuses to take a break. Her strategy? Turning daily chaos into a dance of efficiency and love. She found a rhythm that allowed her to be present for her kids and take care of herself. Her secret weapon was humor, transforming moments of frustration into laughter. A misplaced sock turned into a sock puppet show, and a spill became a chance for a family dance-off. Humor became her shield, protecting her spirit even on the most challenging days.

An athlete's story takes us down a different path. Imagine dedicating your life to sports, only to have an injury change everything. The transition from peak physical condition to chronic pain was jarring, yet it sparked a new journey of adaptation. Through creative expression, like painting and writing, this athlete found healing. Art allowed emotions to flow freely, turning pain into beauty. Each brushstroke became a testament to resilience, a reminder that creativity can flourish even in adversity. Art wasn't just a hobby but a lifeline, offering a new way to process and express experiences that words alone couldn't capture.

Volunteer work and advocacy also offer pathways to resilience. Many individuals have found strength through helping others, even when they're grappling with their own challenges. By engaging in community service, they shift focus from their pain to the impact they can make. Volunteering becomes a powerful tool for building resilience, offering a sense of purpose, and transcending personal struggles. Advocacy, too, plays a role, enabling individuals to fight for change and support others in similar situations. This engagement fosters a sense of belonging and empowerment as they witness the ripple effect of their efforts in the community.

Community-based initiatives further highlight the power of coming together. Local support groups, for example, organize awareness events that educate the public about chronic pain, reduce stigma, and foster understanding. These events are more than informational; they're celebrations of resilience, bringing people together to share stories and support. Online communities offer another avenue, connecting individuals across distances with shared experiences. They create spaces for empathy and encouragement where members can exchange ideas and find solace in knowing they're not alone. These initiatives build support networks, providing invaluable resources and camaraderie for those navigating chronic pain.

From these stories, we learn that adversity often catalyzes personal growth. Patience and empathy become vital companions, teaching individuals to navigate each day gracefully. Once seen as a weakness, vulnerability transforms into a source of strength. Embracing change and adaptability, individuals discover resilience they didn't know they had. They learn to find joy in small victories and to approach setbacks with a renewed perspective. These lessons, born from hardship, illuminate the path forward, guiding individuals to a place where strength and hope intertwine.

Reflection Exercise: Your Resilience Narrative

Take a moment to reflect on your own journey with chronic pain. Consider the strategies that have helped you build resilience. Write down moments where you've found strength and the lessons you've learned along the way. Use this exercise as a reminder of your own capacity to adapt and thrive, even in the face of challenges.

DEVELOPING A PROACTIVE PAIN MANAGEMENT MINDSET

Imagine waking up each day with a fresh sense of purpose, even when chronic pain threatens to cast a shadow. Developing a proactive pain management mindset can transform this vision into reality. It starts with setting goals, but not just any goals—SMART goals, which are Specific, Measurable, Achievable, Relevant, and Time-bound. These aren't just words; they're a framework that helps you focus your efforts and resources efficiently. Instead of a vague aim like "feel better," a SMART goal might be "reduce daily pain levels by practicing mindfulness exercises for 15 minutes each morning for the next month." This gives you a clear target and a timeline, making it easier to track progress. Daily action plans allow you to break down these goals into manageable steps. Like building a puzzle, each piece you fit together is a small victory, bringing the bigger picture into focus. Celebrate these achievements, no matter how small. They are milestones on your path to managing pain effectively.

Self-efficacy is the belief in your ability to control your circumstances, and it's a powerful ally in managing chronic pain. Building this confidence begins with recognizing your strengths and asserting your needs. Start by listing your achievements, no matter how trivial they may seem. Perhaps you attended a social event despite your pain or learned a new coping strategy. Acknowledge these wins and let them fuel your self-belief. Assertiveness is crucial when interacting with healthcare providers. Don't hesitate to ask questions or express concerns. Remember, you're an active participant in your care, not just a bystander. Taking an active role in healthcare decisions means being informed and involved. Research treatment options, seek second opinions if necessary, and trust your instincts. You know your body best, and your voice shapes your treatment plan.

When life throws challenges your way, effective problem-solving techniques are your toolkit for overcoming them. Start by identifying and analyzing the problem at hand. Break it down into smaller components to understand its root causes. This process is like detective work, uncovering clues to guide your next steps. Once you have a clear picture, brainstorm creative solutions. Don't limit yourself to conventional ideas; think outside the box. What worked for someone else might not work for you, and that's okay. Implement your chosen strategy and evaluate its effectiveness. Did it bring relief? If not, keep going. Use this to refine your approach, learning and adapting along the way.

Cultivating a positive and adaptable mindset is the cornerstone of resilience. It's about practicing gratitude and focusing on the positives, even when faced with setbacks. Begin by keeping a gratitude journal, jotting down three daily things you're thankful for. These can be as simple as a sunny morning or a supportive friend. Shifting focus to these positive elements can improve your outlook and reduce stress. When setbacks occur, view them as opportunities for growth. Reframe challenges as learning experiences, asking yourself what they can teach you about your strengths and resilience. Building mental flexibility means being open to change and adjusting your plans. Life is unpredictable, and adaptability is your secret weapon for navigating it.

As you continue your journey with chronic pain, remember that a proactive mindset is not about eliminating pain entirely but managing it effectively. Each small step you take, each goal you achieve, and each problem you solve contributes to a life where pain doesn't control you. This chapter has equipped you with the tools to cultivate self-efficacy, set meaningful goals, and embrace resilience. As we move forward, let's explore how these skills intertwine with community and support, creating a network that sustains and uplifts you.

CHAPTER 18
NAVIGATING SOCIAL INTERACTIONS

Imagine you're at a dinner party, the kind where the host has gone all out with the fancy cutlery and the excellent wine. The conversation flows around you like a river, but you're stuck on the banks, trying to find a way to dive in. Why? Because chronic pain is the elephant in the room, and you need to figure out how to introduce it to everyone without turning the party into an impromptu therapy session. Managing social interactions when you're dealing with chronic pain can feel a bit like learning a new dance—one where the steps aren't always clear, and the rhythm is constantly changing. It's about finding that delicate balance between sharing enough so others understand and not feeling like you're oversharing.

COMMUNICATING PAIN NEEDS TO OTHERS

Let's start with the importance of open communication. It's like having a well-tuned piano. Every key, when pressed, should resonate clearly, creating harmony rather than discord. In relationships, clarity and transparency are your keys. When you share your pain experiences openly, you build a foundation of trust. Friends, family, and colleagues aren't mind readers. They need to understand what you're going through to offer the proper support and accommodations. Imagine trying to bake a cake without a recipe; that's how others might feel. Trying to support you without clear communication and being open sets the stage for stronger bonds, reducing misunderstandings, and fostering empathy.

Effective communication isn't just about speaking; it's about how you talk. Think of it as painting a picture with words. Use descriptive language to convey your pain levels. Instead of saying, "I'm in pain," try, "It feels like there's a heavy weight pressing on my back." This gives others a more vivid understanding of what you're experiencing. Share personal anecdotes to illustrate daily challenges, like how getting out of bed can feel like climbing a mountain on bad days. This not only humanizes your experience but also invites empathy and understanding. Encourage questions. When people ask, they're showing interest and willingness to learn. It opens a dialogue, turning a monologue into a conversation.

Emotional barriers can make open communication feel like a daunting task. Guilt and embarrassment often creep in, whispering that you're burdening others or your pain isn't valid. It's essential to recognize these feelings as obstacles, not truths. Overcoming the fear of judgment or disbelief requires courage and self-compassion. Remember, your pain is real, and your experiences are valid. Initiating difficult conversations can be like standing on the edge of a diving board, hesitant to jump. Start small. Choose a comfortable setting, perhaps over tea or during a walk. Begin with, "I've been wanting to talk about something important to me..." This sets a gentle tone, easing you and the listener into the conversation.

Practical tools can be incredibly helpful in facilitating these conversations. Pain scales or charts can quantify your pain, offering a tangible way for others to grasp its intensity. It's like giving them a map to navigate your experience. Writing letters or emails can be a thoughtful alternative when verbal communication feels overwhelming. They allow you to articulate your thoughts without the pressure of an immediate response. Role-playing scenarios with a trusted friend can also be beneficial. It provides a safe space to practice articulating your needs building confidence for real-life interactions.

Interactive Element: Pain Communication Checklist

Use this checklist to prepare for conversations about your pain:

- Define the Objective: What do you hope to achieve with this conversation? Clarity on this will guide your discussion.
- Choose the Right Time and Place: Select a setting where both parties are comfortable and not rushed.
- Prepare Your Language: Consider using metaphors or analogies to describe your pain.
- Invite Dialogue: Encourage open-ended questions to foster understanding.
- Review Your Boundaries: Know what you're comfortable sharing and where you prefer to draw the line.

Navigating social interactions with chronic pain is an ongoing process. It requires patience, both with yourself and others. Remember, communication is a bridge. It connects you to those who care about you, offering a path toward mutual understanding and support. While it may feel challenging, each conversation is a step toward a more supportive and empathetic environment. A conversation in inspirational stories follows in the next chapter.

CHAPTER 19
INSPIRATIONAL STORIES OF MANAGING CHRONIC PAIN

Picture this: you're at a campfire, stars twinkling above, and someone begins to share a story. Not just any tale, but one that resonates deep within, stirring emotions and sparking insights. That's the power of storytelling, especially regarding chronic pain. It's about weaving narratives that connect us, offering a sense of camaraderie and understanding in our shared experiences. Stories are the threads that bind us, turning solitary struggles into collective courage. They remind us that we're not alone on this path; others have walked it before and found ways to light the way forward.

The real magic of storytelling lies in its ability to foster resilience. When we hear about someone who has faced the relentless storm of chronic pain and emerged with newfound strength, it plants a seed of hope within us. It's like watching someone scale a mountain we've only dared to dream of climbing. We learn from their triumphs, finding inspiration in their perseverance and creativity. As importantly, we know from their setbacks, those moments when the mountain seemed insurmountable. These stories teach us that stumbling and falling is part of the journey and that resilience is born not from avoiding obstacles but from rising to meet them.

Consider Beth Thorp's story, a testament to the transformative power of resilience. Beth, a 59-year-old woman, has been living with chronic pain for about 18 years. Her pain started as left-sided sciatica and expanded to her lower back, neck, arms, and other body parts. But rather than letting the pain define her, Beth focused on what she could do. She embraced movement and exercise, finding solace in walking and low-impact aerobics. She learned that a change of scenery, a breath of fresh air, could work wonders for her spirit. Beth also discovered the power of distraction, immersing herself in books and shows that whisked her mind away from pain's clutches.

Beth's story also highlights the importance of community. She joined support groups and found a network of individuals who truly understood her struggles. Together, they shared insights and encouragement, turning what could have been a solitary battle into a shared experience. This sense of connection is invaluable. It reminds us that while pain may be a constant companion, we don't have to face it alone. Through storytelling, we build a tapestry of experiences, each thread woven with the strength of those who've come before us.

Reflection Section: Craft Your Own Story

Take a moment to reflect on your journey with chronic pain. Consider the challenges you've faced and the victories you've achieved. Write down your story, focusing on your cultivated strength and resilience. Share it with a friend or a support group, or keep it for yourself as a reminder of your courage and growth.

Each story is a testament to your journey, an inspiration to others, and a beacon of hope for yourself.

STAYING MOTIVATED: TURNING SETBACKS INTO STEPPING STONES

Living with chronic pain is like trying to climb a mountain only to find that someone keeps moving the peak further away. No matter how well-prepared you are, setbacks are as inevitable as the sunrise. They're those pesky potholes on the road to recovery; the detours seem to pop up just as you think you've mapped your route. But here's the thing: setbacks are not roadblocks; they're part of the process, a natural ebb and flow in the rhythm of life with chronic pain. Recognizing this can be liberating. It's understanding that progress isn't a straight line but a winding path with peaks and valleys. Each setback is an opportunity to learn, reassess, and gather strength for the next steps. It's about perspective, seeing each challenge not as a failure but as a valuable teacher.

Now, staying motivated when things go sideways is no small feat, but it's doable. One powerful strategy is reframing setbacks as temporary blips on the radar. Instead of dwelling on the immediate frustration, focus on the long-term goals. Picture them as your North Star guiding you through stormy seas. Celebrate small victories along the way; those little wins are the fuel that keeps your engine running. You may have gotten out of bed quicker today or found a new exercise that didn't leave you in agony. These achievements, however minor they seem, deserve recognition. They're the stepping stones that lead to more considerable successes. And when motivation wanes, seek inspiration from role models who exemplify resilience. Whether it's a public figure who has overcome immense odds or someone in your community who radiates positivity, these examples remind us that perseverance pays off.

When setbacks strike, analyzing the situation and planning your recovery is crucial. Ask yourself what factors contributed to the setback. Was it overexertion, stress, or perhaps a change in routine? Identifying these elements helps in developing a strategic plan for bouncing back. Create actionable steps to address these issues, like crafting a to-do list for your recovery. This might involve adjusting your activity level, incorporating more rest periods, or seeking professional guidance. It's about taking control and proactively addressing the factors within your grasp.

Adopting a growth mindset can transform how you perceive setbacks. Embrace challenges as opportunities for development. Every stumble is a chance to learn, to refine your strategies, and to emerge stronger. Self-reflection becomes your compass, guiding you through turbulent times. Assess what worked and didn't, and use these insights to shape future actions. It's not about perfection but progress, understanding that each experience adds a layer to your resilience. With this mindset, setbacks become less daunting and more like stepping stones, leading you to new heights and a greater understanding of your own capabilities.

BALANCING SOCIAL LIFE AND PAIN MANAGEMENT

Living with chronic pain can sometimes feel like you're stuck in a solo act when all you want is to join the ensemble. Yet, maintaining social connections isn't just about having fun; it's vital for your emotional well-being. When you're with others, you tap into a wellspring of emotional support that acts as a buffer against stress. It's like having a safety net that catches you when the tightrope of life gets wobbly. Engaging socially can significantly reduce feelings of isolation and loneliness, reminding you that you're part of a community, not just an island unto yourself. These connections can provide laughter, empathy, and understanding, all potent antidotes to the emotional toll chronic pain can take.

However, planning social activities when managing chronic pain requires a bit of strategy. It's all about knowing your energy peaks and valleys and scheduling activities during prime times. Maybe you're a morning person who feels best after coffee and a good stretch. In that case, brunch dates or morning walks could be your sweet spot. When choosing venues, opt for places with comfortable seating and easy accessibility. Think of it as setting the stage for a successful outing. A cozy café with cushioned chairs or a friend's house where you can kick back might be ideal. And remember, setting time limits for these interactions can help you enjoy them without feeling drained. Use a timer if you have to; there's no shame in bowing out when your body signals it's time for a break.

Managing pain while still enjoying yourself is possible with a few tricks when you're out and about. Portable pain relief tools can be lifesavers. Keep a small heat pack or cushion in your bag when discomfort crashes the party. Scheduled breaks are essential, too. They're like pit stops in a race, allowing you to recharge and continue without burning out. Find a quiet corner or a comfortable resting spot for a few minutes. And don't shy away from practicing discreet stretches or exercises. Maybe it's a gentle neck roll or a subtle leg stretch under the table—whatever helps ease tension without drawing too much attention.

Establishing boundaries is crucial for maintaining your social life without compromising your needs. It starts with learning to say no to overwhelming commitments. It's okay to decline an invitation or reschedule plans if it is too much. Prioritize engagements that are meaningful to you, choosing quality over quantity. Communicating your boundaries clearly to friends and family can prevent misunderstandings and ensure your needs are respected. Let them know what you can handle and what might be too much. This way, you can enjoy social interactions on your terms, creating a balance that supports your well-being and relationships. Social engagement isn't just a luxury; it's a lifeline, offering a sense of belonging and support. The next chapter will consider future directions in pain management.

CHAPTER 20
FUTURE DIRECTIONS IN PAIN MANAGEMENT

Imagine a world where the very concept of pain management has evolved beyond the conventional. This isn't science fiction; it's the cutting edge of research and innovation. Picture a room full of scientists, each armed with a metaphorical paint-brush, working feverishly to color outside the lines of traditional medicine. They're not just tweaking old formulas but creating new canvases of healing. The future is bright—or at least, it's getting there, thanks to groundbreaking developments in pharmacological research, neuromodulation technologies, regenerative medicine, and interdisciplinary collaboration.

Let's start with novel pharmacological breakthroughs. For years, pain management has heavily relied on opioids, often leading to dependency and side effects that make you feel like you're on a roller coaster you didn't pay to ride. But now, researchers are developing non-opioid analgesics that promise to deliver pain relief without the baggage. LSU Health New Orleans, for instance, has created a drug called SRP-001, which is non-addictive and non-toxic. This candidate targets acute and chronic pain, including the thorny issue of migraines, without the organ toxicity or addiction potential of its predecessors. It's already passed Phase 1 human trials, and the FDA has granted it Fast Track designation, which is a bit like giving it a VIP pass to the world of clinical trials. Imagine a pain relief option that doesn't come with a side of guilt or a long list of potential complications. This is the kind of innovation that could redefine how we perceive pain management.

Moving from the realm of chemistry to the electrical highways of our nervous systems, neuromodulation technologies are making waves. If you've ever wished you could just flick a switch to turn down the pain, neuromodulation might be the closest thing to that fantasy. We're talking about devices that can modulate the nerve pathways involved in pain perception. Spinal cord stimulation devices have been around for a while, but new advances make them more precise and effective. Imagine a tiny conductor orchestrating the chaos of nerve signals, turning a cacophony into a symphony. Peripheral nerve stimulation is another promising avenue, focusing on localized pain areas and offering targeted relief without the systemic effects. It's like having a personal pain manager where you need it most.

Regenerative medicine takes a different approach, aiming to heal and rebuild rather than just mask symptoms. Imagine harnessing the power of your own body to repair itself. Researchers are exploring stem cell therapy to regenerate damaged tissues and reduce inflammation. Mesenchymal stem cells, like the Swiss Army knives of the cell world, have shown promise in treating everything from discogenic back pain to osteoarthritis. They can be harvested from your body, reducing the risk of rejection. Then there's platelet-rich plasma (PRP) therapy, which involves injecting a concentration of your own platelets into injured areas to accelerate healing. It's like sending a specialized repair crew to the injury site, equipped with the tools to rebuild.

Interdisciplinary research is the glue that binds all these innovations together. Think of it as a potluck dinner where every guest brings a dish that complements the others. By integrating psychology and neuroscience, researchers better understand how lifestyle factors impact pain. How you think and feel can influence physical sensations and vice versa. This holistic view provides a more comprehensive approach to managing chronic pain, recognizing it as a physiological and psychological experience. Collaborations between disciplines lead to more nuanced treatments that address the whole person, not just the symptoms.

New treatments and technologies are not just about reducing pain but enhancing life quality. They offer hope and possibilities, opening doors that were previously closed. It's an exciting time in pain management, and the innovations on the horizon are as diverse as they are promising.

Interactive Element: Innovations in Pain Management

- Journal Prompt: Reflect on how new treatments like non-opioid analgesics, neuromodulation, or regenerative medicine might change your approach to managing pain. Consider the impact they could have on your daily life and well-being. Write about your hopes and any questions you might have about these innovations.

This bright new world of pain management is still being painted, and while the final picture isn't complete, every new brushstroke brings us closer to a future where pain doesn't hold the brush. The path forward is paved with curiosity, innovation, and a shared commitment to easing the burden of chronic pain.

THE ROLE OF AI IN PAIN MANAGEMENT

Artificial intelligence is revolutionizing the way we approach healthcare, especially in the realm of chronic pain management. Imagine a world where your doctor isn't just a person in a white coat but also a sophisticated AI system equipped with the ability to analyze vast amounts of patient data. This isn't some far-off dream; it's already happening. AI-driven algorithms can now sift through mountains of medical records and patient histories to enhance the accuracy and efficiency of diagnosing chronic pain. These algorithms can identify patterns and correlations that humans might miss, helping doctors pinpoint the source of pain more precisely. Machine learning models are also making strides, predicting treatment outcomes with a level of accuracy that was once unimaginable. By analyzing data from countless patients, these models can suggest which therapies will likely be most effective for your specific condition, potentially saving you time, money, and a lot of trial and error.

But it doesn't stop there. AI is also opening the door to personalized medicine, tailoring treatment plans to fit each patient's unique genetic and biological makeup. Picture this: you're in a doctor's office, and instead of getting a standard prescription, the doctor inputs your genetic profile into an AI system. The system analyzes your data alongside millions of other profiles, recommending a medication dosage specifically for you. It's like having a suit tailored to fit your exact measurements. This level of personalization extends beyond medication. AI can also help identify the best non-pharmacological interventions for you, whether it's acupuncture, physical therapy, or meditation. By considering your entire health profile, AI offers a holistic approach to pain management that feels more like a custom-made plan rather than a one-size-fits-all solution.

AI's role doesn't end with treatment personalization; it also plays a critical role in pain tracking and monitoring. Wearable sensors powered by AI are becoming more common, providing real-time data on pain metrics. Imagine wearing a device that tracks your heart rate and steps and monitors your pain levels throughout the day. These sensors can alert you to changes that might predict a flare-up, helping you take proactive measures to manage your pain. AI applications also automate pain diary entries, transforming the tedious task of logging symptoms into a seamless process. This automation saves time and ensures more accurate data collection, benefiting both you and your healthcare provider. Furthermore, predictive analytics use this data to anticipate pain episodes before they happen, allowing you to adjust your activities and medications accordingly. It's like having a weather forecast for your body, helping you prepare for stormy days.

Yet, as with any powerful tool, integrating AI into pain management comes with ethical considerations and challenges. One primary concern is data privacy and patient consent. When dealing with sensitive health information, protecting your data is paramount. Patients must clearly understand how their data will be used and can opt-out. Another challenge is providing equitable access to AI-driven healthcare tools. Some people have different access to technology, and AI could widen the gap between those who can afford these advanced tools and those who cannot. These innovations must remain accessible to all, regardless of socioeconomic status. Additionally, there are concerns about algorithmic bias, where AI systems may inadvertently favor specific demographics over others. We must address these issues head-on, ensuring that AI in pain management is fair, transparent, and beneficial for everyone.

The integration of AI into pain management is a promising development that holds the potential to transform how we understand

and treat chronic pain. From improving diagnostic accuracy to tailoring personalized treatment plans and enhancing monitoring systems, AI brings a wealth of opportunities. However, as we embrace these advancements, we must remain vigilant about ethical considerations, ensuring all patients benefit from these technologies. The future of pain management is undoubtedly exciting, but it requires careful navigation to ensure that innovation aligns with equity and empathy. In the next chapter, we will explore how the role of the caregiver works hand in hand for better patient outcomes.

CHAPTER 21
ROLE OF THE CAREGIVER

Imagine yourself as an orchestra conductor, where each instrument represents a different aspect of your life. Your caregiver, whether a family member, friend, or healthcare professional, plays the role of the first violin, helping maintain harmony amidst chronic pain's cacophony. Their support is invaluable, but like any great symphony, it requires clear communication to ensure each note is played in tune. In the realm of chronic pain management, effective communication with caregivers is not merely beneficial—it's essential. Through this dialogue, you can articulate your needs, share the nuances of your pain, and build a partnership that thrives on empathy and understanding.

Understanding the dynamics of caregiver-patient communication is akin to learning a new language. It's about more than just speaking; it's about listening actively and recognizing the symphony of non-verbal cues accompanying words. When your caregiver truly listens, they tune into the subtleties of your experience, picking up on the unspoken signals that words often fail to convey. A nod or a soft touch can express understanding. At the same time, a furrowed brow might indicate confusion. By being attentive to these signals, communication becomes a two-way street, where both parties feel heard and validated. This mutual understanding forms the bedrock of a supportive relationship that can weather the storms of chronic pain.

Yet, even in the best circumstances, communication barriers can arise, like static on a radio. Misinterpretation of pain levels is a common challenge. What feels like a gentle wave to you might seem like a tidal wave to your caregiver. Emotional fatigue can also cloud interactions, making it challenging to articulate needs clearly. Both you and your caregiver might feel overwhelmed by the relentless nature of chronic pain, leading to misunderstandings and frustration. Recognizing these barriers is the first step toward dismantling them, allowing for more transparent and effective communication.

To improve communication skills, consider adopting practical strategies that foster understanding and connection. Using "I" statements to express your needs and feelings can be a game changer. Instead of saying, "You don't understand my pain," try, "I feel overwhelmed when my pain isn't acknowledged." This subtle shift focuses on your experience, reducing defensiveness and inviting empathy. Regular check-ins can also strengthen the caregiver-patient bond. Set aside time to discuss pain management progress, celebrate small victories, and address concerns. This consistent dialogue nurtures trust and keeps both parties aligned in their goals.

Setting clear boundaries and expectations is another vital component of effective communication. Defining what you need from your caregiver and what you can manage independently is essential. This clarity helps prevent misunderstandings and empowers you and your caregiver to fulfill your roles effectively. Remember, boundaries are not walls but guidelines for maintaining a healthy and balanced relationship.

Incorporating communication aids into your routine can further enhance understanding and collaboration. Pain diaries, for instance, serve as tangible records of your daily experiences, helping you track symptoms and identify patterns. Sharing this information with your caregiver gives them a clearer picture of your journey, facilitating more informed discussions. Technology aids, like shared medication tracking apps, ensure that you and your caregiver are on the same page regarding treatment regimens. These tools act as bridges, connecting your experiences and insights with their support and expertise.

Interactive Element: Communication Checklist

Consider creating a communication checklist to guide your interactions with your caregiver. Include items such as "Share daily pain levels," "Discuss any new symptoms," and "Review treatment plan adjustments." Use this checklist during your regular check-ins to ensure all essential topics are covered. It's a simple yet powerful tool to keep communication flowing smoothly and prevent critical details from slipping through the cracks.

Navigating the caregiver-patient relationship is a journey of shared experiences and mutual growth. You create a supportive environment where you and your caregiver can thrive by fostering open communication, recognizing barriers, and employing strategies and tools to enhance dialogue. In this symbiotic dance, you are not alone; you have a partner who stands by your side, ready to support you in facing the challenges of chronic pain.

BUILDING A SUPPORTIVE ENVIRONMENT

Imagine your life as a puzzle, each representing a different aspect of support: family, friends, healthcare professionals, and your physical space. When these pieces fit together, they form a picture of resilience and strength, providing a foundation to manage chronic pain effectively. A holistic support system doesn't just enhance your physical health; it nurtures your emotional well-being too. Family and friends offer a shoulder to lean on, a listening ear, and the encouragement you need on tough days. They help transform isolation into connection, reducing the burden of chronic pain. Meanwhile, healthcare professionals bring expertise and guidance, ensuring your treatment plan is tailored to your needs. This collaboration creates a safety net that catches you when the going gets tough, offering reassurance that you're not alone in this.

Your home environment plays a crucial role in this support system. It's your sanctuary, where you should feel safe and comfortable. By optimizing your living space, you can reduce the physical strain of daily activities. Simple changes, like rearranging furniture to create clear pathways, can significantly minimize movement strain. Consider the placement of frequently used items; keeping them within easy reach can prevent unnecessary bending or stretching. Assistive devices and tools, like grab bars in the bathroom or a reacher for high shelves, can further enhance accessibility, allowing you to maintain independence while managing pain. These modifications create an environment that supports your physical needs and fosters a sense of control over your surroundings.

Emotional and psychological support practices are equally vital. They form the glue that holds your support system together, promoting resilience and well-being for both you and your caregiver. Joint stress-relief activities, like mindfulness or meditation, offer moments of peace amidst the chaos of chronic pain. These practices encourage relaxation, reduce stress, and strengthen the bond between you and your caregiver. Family therapy sessions can also be beneficial, providing a space to address emotional challenges, improve communication, and develop strategies for coping as a unit. These shared experiences foster understanding and empathy, reinforcing that you're in this together.

While the focus often lies on the person experiencing chronic pain, it's essential to acknowledge the well-being of the caregiver, too. Their role is demanding, and their health is crucial for adequate support. Encourage your caregiver to prioritize self-care routines that replenish their energy and resilience. Whether it's a daily walk, a hobby they love, or simply taking time to relax, these activities are vital for their well-being. Managing caregiver burnout is another critical consideration. Burnout can manifest as physical exhaustion, emotional fatigue, or helplessness. Encourage your caregiver to recognize these signs and seek support through therapy, support groups, or simply talking with friends. Accessing caregiver support groups can provide a valuable outlet for sharing experiences, gaining insights, and finding encouragement from others in similar roles.

In this intricate dance of support, each person plays a vital role. Family, friends, healthcare providers, and caregivers form a network that sustains you through the challenges of chronic pain. By nurturing these relationships, optimizing your environment, and prioritizing emotional resilience, you create a supportive ecosystem that bolsters your physical health and emotional well-being. As you continue to navigate the complexities of chronic pain, remember that this support system is your ally, always ready to lift you up and help you move forward toward turning pain to power.

CHAPTER 22
PAIN TO POWER

EMBRACE THE PAIN AS A TEACHER

Imagine your pain as a quirky old professor with a penchant for surprises—with a habit of turning up uninvited to deliver life's most profound lessons. While it may not have the charm of a favorite teacher, it brings wisdom that only experience can offer. Each ache and struggle becomes a chapter in your personal guidebook, showing you what truly matters. Pain has a way of stripping life down to its essentials. It's like pruning a garden, removing the weeds to let the flowers thrive. It forces you to re-evaluate priorities to see where your energy is best spent. When you view pain as a teacher, you learn to listen to your body and mind, discovering a resilience you might not have known you possessed.

As you navigate this educational journey, take note of the insights that surface. You may find that patience becomes your ally, or empathy for others grows as you understand their hidden battles. Pain teaches you to appreciate the good days and to find joy in small victories. Over time, it urges you to let go of what no longer serves you, making room for growth and transformation. No one would choose this lesson, but once you're in the classroom, the lessons are invaluable. Each moment of discomfort can lead to a deeper understanding of yourself, revealing strengths and capacities you never imagined. Embracing pain as a teacher can empower you to face life's challenges with grace and humor, finding meaning and purpose even amid adversity.

Reflection Section: Journaling Prompt

Write about a time when your pain taught you something about yourself. What did you learn, and how did it change your perspective? Use this exercise to uncover the hidden gifts within your experiences, turning pain into a source of wisdom.

SHIFT FOCUS FROM SUFFERING TO RESILIENCE

Every morning when you rise, no matter how stiff or sore, you're not just getting out of bed—you're staking a claim on your own resilience. It's like facing a storm with nothing but an umbrella and a can-do attitude. You're not pretending the storm isn't there, but you're also not letting it sweep you away. Each day you choose to face discomfort with courage, you're building a fortress of strength, brick by brick. It's not about denying the pain but recognizing the power you hold to keep moving forward. This isn't a sprint; it's a marathon, and every step you take is a testament to your determination.

Think of resilience as your secret superpower, which develops quietly, often unnoticed, until needed. It's the ability to adapt and find new ways to thrive even when things go sideways. You might not have chosen this path, but here you are, navigating it with grit you didn't know you had. Each challenge met, and each hurdle overcome adds to your inner strength. It's like weightlifting for the soul. And just like with any exercise, the more you practice resilience, the stronger it gets. The beauty of this strength is that it extends beyond physical pain—it touches every area of your life. It influences how you tackle challenges at work, support friends, and approach life's uncertainties. Every day you're faced with discomfort, you're also allowed to rise above it, to prove to yourself that you are capable, no matter what. So when the alarm rings and your joints protest, remember: resilience isn't just about enduring—it's about living fully despite everything.

TRANSFORM EMOTIONAL ENERGY INTO PURPOSE

With all its weight and intensity, pain can become a powerful energy source, much like the heat that powers a steam engine. It's there; it demands attention, and if you harness it wisely, it can propel you forward. When you focus this energy on something meaningful, it's as if you're turning pain into a different kind of fuel—something that ignites passion, creativity, and drive. Whether volunteering at a local shelter, painting a canvas with colors that reflect your emotions, or writing a blog to share your story, these actions give purpose to the pain. They transform the narrative from one of suffering to one of creation. Imagine your pain as the clay on a potter's wheel. It starts as a lump, unformed and heavy, but with each turn and touch, it shapes into something beautiful and unique. This is the essence of channeling emotional energy into purpose. Your pain becomes a tool for shaping your world, for building something that resonates with your values and passions.

Consider the moments when you've felt the most alive, even if they were fleeting. Those times when you lost track of the hours because you were so engrossed in what you were doing. That's the kind of purpose that transforms. It's the kind that lets you forget about the pain, even if just for a little while, and enables you to focus on what you love. It's about finding those activities that make your heart sing and diving into them with all your might. You'll find that these pursuits distract from the pain and provide a sense of accomplishment and fulfillment.

FIND GROWTH IN EACH CHALLENGE

When faced with pain, it's easy to focus on what's being taken from you. Yet, beneath the surface, something profound is happening. Each challenge is like a sculptor's chisel, slowly revealing the masterpiece within. As you navigate these obstacles, you might notice a shift. Questions arise: "What can I learn from this?" "How can this experience mold me into someone stronger?" In answering these, you discover that your pain lays a sturdy foundation built on empathy, patience, and grit. Empathy grows as you understand the silent battles others might be fighting. You find yourself offering a listening ear or a comforting word, something you might have overlooked. Patience becomes more than just a virtue; it's a survival skill. It teaches you to wait, endure, and find peace amidst chaos. Grit, however, is the real game changer. It's the determination to keep moving forward, even when every step feels like wading through mud. Each setback, every moment of discomfort, becomes a step forward, a lesson in resilience and adaptability.

These qualities don't just appear overnight. They develop slowly, like a muscle, growing stronger with each repetition. Over time, you realize that your unwelcome pain has been your most outstanding teacher in disguise. It equips you with tools to face the future and handle whatever comes next with newfound strength. In the quiet moments, when you reflect on your journey, you'll see the growth. The person you were is not the person you are now.

You've changed, adapted, and become someone who can weather any storm with grace and courage.

RECLAIM YOUR STORY

Picture yourself standing at a crossroads. On one side, there's the familiar path of victimhood—a road worn down by repeated tales of defeat and hardship. But look closer; you'll see another less traveled path where the narrative is entirely yours to create. This is where you reclaim your story. It's about changing the script from one dictated by pain to one where you are the author. In this version, you're not defined by what you've lost but by how you've risen. Here, you are a warrior who faces battles daily, armed with grit, determination, and a spirit that refuses to be subdued.

Reclaiming your story means acknowledging your pain without allowing it to overshadow your identity. It's about embracing the power to redefine your life, even if it means starting with small victories. It's as simple as finding joy in a hobby you had set aside or reaching out to others who understand your experience. No matter how small, each step you take is a rewrite of the narrative. You are not just surviving—you are thriving, crafting a life that celebrates your victories, however minor they may seem. This path is about empowerment, recognizing that pain is part of your story but doesn't hold the pen. You do. And with it, you write chapters filled with resilience, courage, and hope. As you reclaim your story, remember that every page turned is a testament to a life lived fully, even amidst challenges. As we transition to the next chapter, we'll explore financial considerations when dealing with chronic pain.

CHAPTER 23
FINANCIAL CONSIDERATIONS

Imagine this: you're the star of a thrilling action movie where chronic pain is the villain, and your wallet is the trusty sidekick. You need to fend off those daring medical bills without sacrificing your financial sanity. The good news is you don't need to be a financial guru or a superhero to find ways to manage costs effectively. We're diving into the world of cost-effective treatment options, where every penny saved is a victory over chronic pain. We'll explore affordable medication alternatives, community resources, home-based remedies, and government assistance programs. These strategies will empower you to make informed decisions while keeping your budget intact.

COST-EFFECTIVE TREATMENT OPTIONS

Let's start with affordable medication alternatives. Did you know that choosing generic drugs over brand-name ones can save you a small fortune? They're like the store-brand cereal that tastes just as good as the name-brand stuff but at half the price. Generics contain the same active ingredients, ensuring you get the relief you need without the premium cost. Over-the-counter (OTC) options like acetaminophen and ibuprofen are also great allies in the battle against pain. They're readily available, budget-friendly, and can be just as effective for many types of pain. These OTC medications are the unsung heroes of pain relief, always there for you when you need them, like a trusty friend who never lets you down.

Community and non-profit resources are like hidden gems in the treasure chest of pain management. Local clinics often operate on a sliding scale, ensuring you only pay what you can afford. These clinics understand that your financial situation shouldn't dictate your access to care. Additionally, non-profit organizations frequently offer free therapy sessions to help those in need. These resources are vital when your financial situation feels as tight as your favorite pair of jeans after the holidays. With some research, you can find programs and organizations that align with your needs, providing relief without the financial strain.

Home-based treatments and self-care practices are the secret weapons in your cost-saving arsenal. You don't need to spend a fortune on fancy gadgets or treatments when you can use simple household items to your advantage. Hot and cold packs, for instance, are a cost-effective way to manage pain. A bag of frozen peas or a warm towel can work wonders on sore muscles and joints. Plenty of online resources offer guided exercises and meditation routines for those who enjoy a bit of DIY. These virtual guides can help you maintain your physical and mental well-being without spending a dime. It's like having a personal trainer and therapist in your living room.

Sometimes, navigating the world of government assistance programs feels like deciphering an ancient map. But fear not—Medicaid and Medicare are there to provide a helping hand. These programs offer various benefits for pain management, depending on your location. Medicaid is beneficial for low-income individuals, while Medicare caters to those over 65 or with specific disabilities. These programs can cover a range of services, from physical therapy to prescription medications. Social Security Disability Benefits may also be available for chronic pain sufferers, offering financial support when work becomes challenging. Understanding these programs and their offerings can be a game-changer, ensuring you get the care you need without breaking the bank.

Interactive Element: Resource Checklist

To make this journey more manageable, consider using a resource checklist. This tool can help you keep track of local clinics, nonprofit organizations, and government programs available in your area. Include contact information, services offered, and any eligibility criteria. Having this information organized and accessible will save you time and stress when you need to reach out for support. Think of it as your personal treasure map, guiding you to the resources you need to navigate the financial challenges of managing chronic pain.

NAVIGATING INSURANCE FOR PAIN MANAGEMENT

Dealing with insurance can feel like trying to solve a Rubik's cube blindfolded. But, understanding the basics of health insurance coverage is the first step in making this daunting task manageable. Let's break down some standard terms you'll encounter. Start with deductibles, the amount you pay out of pocket before your insurance kicks in. Think of it as the cover charge to get inside the club where your benefits are hanging out. Then there are copayments, the flat fees you pay for certain services, like visiting the doctor or getting prescriptions. They're like the appetizer prices at a fancy restaurant—necessary but sometimes surprising. Lastly, out-of-pocket limits cap what you pay annually, protecting you from financial free fall. Understanding these terms will help you navigate the insurance maze and make informed decisions about your coverage.

Regarding prescription medications, coverage can vary widely depending on your plan. Some insurance policies cover a broad range of drugs, while others are more selective, akin to a picky eater at a buffet. Familiarize yourself with your plan's formulary a list of covered drugs, and know which tier your medications fall into. Higher-tier drugs often come with higher costs, so knowing your options can save you money. If your prescribed medication isn't covered, don't despair. Talk to your doctor about alternatives or request a formulary exception from your insurer. It might take some persistence, but advocating for yourself is critical.

Maximizing your insurance benefits requires strategic planning. Choosing a plan with robust pain management coverage is crucial. When shopping for insurance, look for plans that cover a wide range of treatments, from physical therapy to alternative therapies like acupuncture. Annual plan reviews are equally important. Our lives and health needs change, and so should our insurance plans. Make adjustments as necessary to ensure your coverage aligns with your current needs. It's like getting a seasonal wardrobe update—essential for staying prepared and comfortable.

Navigating the challenges of insurance can be frustrating, especially for chronic pain patients. Denial of claims for alternative treatments is a common hurdle. Insurers often stick to conventional treatments, leaving you to argue the merits of your chosen therapy. Persistence is your best ally here. Gather evidence, perhaps studies supporting the efficacy of your treatment, and present it to your insurer. Pre-authorization requirements for procedures are another obstacle. These are like permission slips you need before getting treatment. Work closely with your healthcare provider to ensure all necessary paperwork is submitted accurately and on time. Coverage gaps for chronic conditions can also occur, leaving you without essential care. In these cases, explore supplemental insurance options or financial assistance programs to fill the void.

Effective communication with insurers can feel like navigating a minefield. Start by preparing thorough documentation and medical records for any claims you submit. The more organized and comprehensive your information, the stronger your case. Role-playing phone conversations with insurers can boost your confidence and improve your negotiation skills. Practice explaining your situation clearly and assertively, anticipating potential questions or objections. When claims are denied, writing an effective appeal letter is crucial. Be concise but thorough, explaining why the treatment is necessary and how it benefits your condition. Include supporting documents, such as letters from your healthcare provider and any relevant medical research.

In closing, navigating insurance for pain management can be a labyrinth of terms, conditions, and paperwork. Understanding the basics of coverage, maximizing benefits, overcoming challenges, and effectively communicating with insurers are all part of this complex dance. These strategies can help you make the most of your insurance plan, ensuring you receive the care you need without undue stress or financial strain. As we continue on this journey, remember that knowledge is power, and with a bit of persistence, you can turn the insurance maze into a straightforward path to the treatment you deserve.

CONCLUSION

As we end our journey together, I want to reflect on all we've explored. Chronic pain is a formidable adversary, but understanding it is the first step in reclaiming your life. We've journeyed through the neuroscience of pain, uncovering how it sends electric signals to our brains, rewiring pathways like a renegade electrician. We've talked about the profound impact chronic pain has on mental health, transforming daily life into a roller coaster ride of emotions. We've delved into the myriad of coping mechanisms, from innovative treatments like ketamine infusions and low-dose naltrexone to holistic strategies like mindfulness, meditation, and even embracing humor for resilience.

Throughout this journey, we've emphasized caregivers' vital roles, offering support and strength when needed. We've discussed ergonomic solutions for chronic back pain, turning household chores into manageable tasks rather than daunting endeavors. Mindfulness and meditation have emerged as allies in pain management, providing moments of calm in the storm.

If there's one thing I hope you take away, it's the power of combining medical treatments with holistic approaches. Just as important is the realization that mental health care must walk hand-in-hand with physical pain management. Building a robust and supportive network isn't just beneficial—it's essential. Emerging treatments and technologies, like artificial intelligence, hold promise for advancing pain management and offer hope for a future where pain doesn't dictate our lives.

But remember, managing chronic pain is not just about treatments and techniques. It's a journey, one that demands resilience and proactive engagement. There will be days when pain feels like a relentless tide, but there are also moments of improvement, of strength found in community and self-advocacy. This book is a stepping stone, a guide to inspire hope and empowerment as you navigate your path.

Please take the strategies and insights we've shared and implement them in your life. Start with simple changes in your daily routine, seek out supportive communities, and explore new treatment options. Advocate for your needs in healthcare settings because your voice matters. Continue educating yourself—knowledge is power and your ally in this battle.

On a personal note, as someone who has walked this path, I know how isolating chronic pain can feel. My own journey began with a neck injury in Iraq and has taken me through the complex landscape of complex regional pain syndrome. But it has also brought me here, to this point, sharing with you. I am grateful for your company on this journey and for your courage to face chronic pain head-on. Together, we form a community of resilience and strength.

Let's keep this conversation going. Stay connected through online platforms and support groups. Share your stories and insights because every voice adds to the collective strength of our community. I appreciate your time and commitment to understanding and managing chronic pain. It takes courage to confront pain and resilience to strive for improvement. I commend you for both.

As we close this chapter, I leave you with a hopeful and uplifting message: Empowerment is within your grasp. Despite chronic pain, a fulfilling life is possible. See your journey as one of personal growth and transformation. Each step forward, no matter how small, is a victory. Remember, you are not alone. Together, we can turn pain into power and power into a life lived fully and purposefully.

I hope you found "Pain to Power" helpful! If you found any part of it meaningful or helpful, would you be willing to share your thoughts in a review? Thank you for considering it!

REFERENCES

Central sensitisation in chronic pain conditions https://www.thelancet.com/journals/lanrhe/article/PIIS2665-9913(21)00032-1/fulltext

Chronic pain: The role of learning and brain plasticity - PMC https://pmc.ncbi.nlm.nih.gov/articles/PMC4922795/

Nociceptive and neuropathic pain: What's the difference? https://www.medicalnewstoday.com/articles/319895

Neuroimaging Studies of Chronic Pain - PMC https://pmc.ncbi.nlm.nih.gov/articles/PMC2935976/

Pain and depression: Is there a link? https://www.mayoclinic.org/diseases-conditions/depression/expert-answers/pain-and-depression/faq-20057823

Cognitive Behavioral Therapy for Chronic Pain https://www.va.gov/painmanagement/docs/cbt-cp_therapist_manual.pdf

Ketamine Infusion Therapy and its Role in Chronic Pain https://www.asra.com/news-publications/asra-newsletter/newsletter-item/asra-news/2022/07/29/ketamine-infusion-therapy-and-its-role-in-chronic-pain

Low-Dose Naltrexone (LDN) for Chronic Pain at a Single ... https://www.ncbi.nlm.nih.gov/pmc/articles/PMC10276990/

Mechanisms behind the Development of Chronic Low Back ... https://www.mdpi.com/2075-1729/13/1/84

Mindfulness meditation to control pain https://www.health.harvard.edu/pain/mindfulness-meditation-to-control-pain

The 10 Best Yoga Poses for Back Pain https://www.healthline.com/health/fitness-exercise/yoga-for-back-pain

Treating Chronic Pain With Meditation https://www.theatlantic.com/health/archive/2014/04/treating-chronic-pain-with-meditation/284182/

Complex regional pain syndrome - Symptoms & causes https://www.mayoclinic.org/diseases-conditions/crps-complex-regional-pain-syndrome/symptoms-causes/syc-20371151

Ketamine for Complex Regional Pain Syndrome https://www.ncbi.nlm.nih.gov/pmc/articles/PMC10688501/

Multidisciplinary Management of Complex Regional Pain ... https://pmc.ncbi.nlm.nih.gov/articles/PMC10166377/

Alternative Therapies https://www.burningnightscrps.org/crps/crps-information/crps-treatments/alternative-therapies/

Fibromyalgia - Symptoms & causes https://www.mayoclinic.org/diseases-conditions/fibromyalgia/symptoms-causes/syc-20354780

10 best apps for people with chronic pain https://uspainfoundation.org/blog/10-best-apps-for-people-with-chronic-pain/

Fibromyalgia care https://account.allinahealth.org/services/945

Fibromyalgia and Stress: Understanding the Connection https://www.healthline.com/health/fibromyalgia/fibromyalgia-and-stress

Low-Dose Naltrexone (LDN) for Chronic Pain at a Single ... https://www.ncbi.nlm.nih.gov/pmc/articles/PMC10276990/

Ketamine in Acute and Chronic Pain Management https://www.ncbi.nlm.nih.gov/books/NBK539824/

How Can Biofeedback Therapy Help Chronic Pain? https://www.everydayhealth.com/chronic-pain/biofeedback-therapy-can-help-chronic-pain/

Medicinal Cannabis for Treatment of Chronic Pain https://www.ncbi.nlm.nih.gov/books/NBK574562/

Chronic Pain and Complementary Health Approaches https://www.nccih.nih.gov/health/chronic-pain-and-complementary-health-approaches-usefulness-and-safety

Spirituality Assessments and Interventions In Pain Medicine https://www.medcentral.com/pain/chronic/spirituality-assessments-interventions-pain-medicine

Research Finds Acupuncture Effective for Chronic Pain https://www.aafp.org/news/health-of-the-public/20180521acupuncture.html

Efficacy of Topical Essential Oils in Musculoskeletal ... https://www.ncbi.nlm.nih.gov/pmc/articles/PMC9959659/

10 best apps for people with chronic pain https://uspainfoundation.org/blog/10-best-apps-for-people-with-chronic-pain/

Ergonomics and Chronic Pain https://www.painscale.com/article/ergonomics-and-chronic-pain

7 Exercises for Reducing Chronic Pain https://www.healthline.com/health/exercises-to-reduce-chronic-pain

Mindfulness meditation-based pain relief: a mechanistic ... https://www.ncbi.nlm.nih.gov/pmc/articles/PMC4941786/

5 Tips for Choosing a Pain Management Doctor https://www.psadocs.com/5-tips-for-choosing-a-pain-management-doctor/

Benefits of a Multidisciplinary Approach to Pain Management https://integrativespineandsports.com/exploring-the-benefits-of-a-multidisciplinary-approach-to-pain-management/

6 Chronic Pain Support Groups of 2023 https://www.verywellhealth.com/best-chronic-pain-support-groups-4845866

Resources https://uspainfoundation.org/resources/

The effect of an anti-inflammatory diet on chronic pain https://www.ncbi.nlm.nih.gov/pmc/articles/PMC10381948/

Pain regulation by gut microbiota: molecular mechanisms ... https://www.sciencedirect.com/science/article/pii/S0007091219306385

The anti-inflammatory effects of a Mediterranean diet https://pubmed.ncbi.nlm.nih.gov/36039924/

Eating your way out of pain: How your gut microbiota and diet ... https://www.news-medical.net/news/20230828/Eating-your-way-out-of-pain-How-your-gut-microbiota-and-diet-can-help-manage-chronic-discomfort.aspx

10 best apps for people with chronic pain https://uspainfoundation.org/blog/10-best-apps-for-people-with-chronic-pain/

Innovations in Wearable Technology for Pain ... https://santarosapainandperformance.com/innovations-in-wearable-technology-for-pain-management-and-performance/

Can Virtual Reality Help Ease Chronic Pain? https://www.nytimes.com/2022/04/26/magazine/virtual-reality-chronic-pain.html

Use and efficacy of virtual, augmented, or mixed reality ... https://www.ncbi.nlm.nih.gov/pmc/articles/PMC9517958/

Physical activity and exercise for chronic pain in adults https://pmc.ncbi.nlm.nih.gov/articles/PMC5461882/

Tai Chi for Arthritis: Is It a Good Idea? https://www.healthline.com/health/fitness/tai-chi-for-arthritis

What Is the Spoon Theory Metaphor for Chronic Illness? https://health.clevelandclinic.org/spoon-theory-chronic-illness

Pacing: A concept analysis of a chronic pain intervention https://www.ncbi.nlm.nih.gov/pmc/articles/PMC3812193/

Use mindfulness to cope with chronic pain https://www.mayoclinichealthsystem.org/hometown-health/speaking-of-health/use-mindfulness-to-cope-with-chronic-pain

Body scan mindfulness exercise for pain https://www.health.harvard.edu/pain/body-scan-for-pain

The Effectiveness of Mindfulness-Based Stress Reduction ... https://www.ncbi.nlm.nih.gov/pmc/articles/PMC4873598/

Cognitive-Behavioral Therapy for Individuals with Chronic Pain https://pubmed.ncbi.nlm.nih.gov/24547801/

How Can Biofeedback Therapy Help Chronic Pain? https://www.everydayhealth.com/chronic-pain/biofeedback-therapy-can-help-chronic-pain/

Efficacy of EMG- and EEG-Biofeedback in Fibromyalgia ... https://pmc.ncbi.nlm.nih.gov/articles/PMC3776543

Efficacy of Biofeedback in Chronic Back Pain: a Meta- ... https://pubmed.ncbi.nlm.nih.gov/27307013/

How Can Biofeedback Therapy Help Chronic Pain? https://www.everydayhealth.com/chronic-pain/biofeedback-therapy-can-help-chronic-pain/

8 Myths and Facts About Chronic Pain https://www.webmd.com/pain-management/ss/slideshow-chronic-pain-myths-facts

Unusual Symptoms of Fibromyalgia https://painconsults.com/unusual-symptoms-of-fibromyalgia/

Panel cites need for individualized, patient-centered ... https://www.nih.gov/news-events/news-releases/panel-cites-need-individualized-patient-centered-approach-treat-monitor-chronic-pain

National Pain Advocacy Center https://nationalpain.org/

Sleep deficiency and chronic pain: potential underlying ... https://www.ncbi.nlm.nih.gov/pmc/articles/PMC6879497/

Caffeine Effects on Sleep Taken 0, 3, or 6 Hours before Going ... https://jcsm.aasm.org/doi/10.5664/jcsm.3170

How to Use Meditation for Better Sleep https://www.healthline.com/health/meditation-for-sleep

Chronic Pain and Insomnia: Breaking the Cycle https://www.spine-health.com/wellness/sleep/chronic-pain-and-insomnia-breaking-cycle

Resilience: A New Paradigm for Adaptation to Chronic Pain https://pmc.ncbi.nlm.nih.gov/articles/PMC4899321/

Ketamine: A Rising Star in Mental Health Treatment https://adaa.org/learn-from-us/from-the-experts/blog-posts/consumer-professional/ketamine-rising-star-mental-health

The Role of Support Groups in Pain Management: Finding ... https://www.advancedphysicalmedicinepc.com/post/the-role-of-support-groups-in-pain-management-finding-community-and-empowerment

The Safety and Efficacy of Low-Dose Naltrexone in ... https://pmc.ncbi.nlm.nih.gov/articles/PMC10039621/

Effective Communication Strategies That Help With ... https://www.baltimoretherapycenter.com/effective-communication-strategies-for-chronic-pain/

Overcoming Barriers to Effective Pain Management https://totalpaincarenj.com/wp/2024/03/11/overcoming-barriers-to-effective-pain-management/

Pain Communication Tools https://geriatricpain.org/pain-communication-tools

Interventions to Support Family Caregivers in Pain Management https://pmc.ncbi.nlm.nih.gov/articles/PMC7483228

Living With, and Managing, Chronic Pain: A Patient's Story https://www.medcentral.com/pain/chronic/living-managing-chronic-pain-patient-story

Resilience: A New Paradigm for Adaptation to Chronic Pain https://pmc.ncbi.nlm.nih.gov/articles/PMC4899321/

The healing others: the essential role of social support on ... https://www.ncbi.nlm.nih.gov/pmc/articles/PMC11220379/

Tips to stay motivated with chronic pain https://www.burningnightscrps.org/support/news-and-blog/article/tips-to-stay-motivated-with-chronic-pain/

Novel Non-Addictive, Non-Toxic Painkiller Developed at ... https://www.lsuhsc.edu/news/novel-non-addictive-non-toxic-painkiller-lsu-health-new-orleans.aspx

Neuromodulation techniques – From non-invasive brain ... https://www.sciencedirect.com/science/article/pii/S1878747924000163

Stem Cell Therapy and Its Significance in Pain Management https://pmc.ncbi.nlm.nih.gov/articles/PMC8445610/

Reviewing the Potential Role of Artificial Intelligence in ... https://pmc.ncbi.nlm.nih.gov/articles/PMC10924768/

Effective Communication In Chronic Pain Management https://oklahomapaintreatmentcenters.com/article/effective-communication-in-chronic-pain-management

The Effect of Caregiver-Facilitated Pain Management ... https://www.sciencedirect.com/science/article/pii/S0885392420305741

Factors influencing caregiver burden in chronic pain patients https://pmc.ncbi.nlm.nih.gov/articles/PMC9524903/

How Assistive Devices Help Chronic Pain Management https://healthmaxphysio.com/how-assistive-devices-help-chronic-pain-management/

Ketamine Infusions for Chronic Pain: A Systematic Review... https://journals.lww.com/anesthesia-analgesia/fulltext/2019/07000/ketamine_infusions_for_chronic_pain__a_systematic.40.aspx

Family Caregiver Challenges in Pain Management for ... https://www.ncbi.nlm.nih.gov/pmc/articles/PMC9784612/

Low-dose naltrexone for the treatment of fibromyalgia https://pmc.ncbi.nlm.nih.gov/articles/PMC8591911/

Complex Regional Pain Syndrome (CRPS) https://my.clevelandclinic.org/health/diseases/12085-complex-regional-pain-syndrome-crps

Nonopioid Therapies for Pain Management https://www.cdc.gov/overdose-prevention/hcp/clinical-care/nonopioid-therapies-for-pain-management.html

Living with Pain Resources https://www.iasp-pain.org/resources/living-with-pain/

8 non-invasive pain relief techniques that really work https://www.health.harvard.edu/pain/8-non-invasive-pain-relief-techniques-that-really-work

Do Medicare And Medicaid Cover Pain Management? https://paintherapycare.com/do-medicare-and-medicaid-cover-pain-management/

ABOUT THE AUTHOR

Col (Ret) Strand has been living with chronic pain and advocating for others since he sustained a neck injury in a duty-related accident in Iraq in 2005. Following that, he suffered a broken leg, which led to complications, including Chronic Regional Pain Syndrome (CRPS), often referred to as the "suicide disease" due to its extreme pain. He manages a Facebook group for military personnel and veterans with RSD/CRPS providing ongoing support to help them navigate the disability process. With 34 years of active duty, Col (R) Strand has served as a medical service technician and as an operations officer in four war zones: Saudi Arabia, Bosnia, the Republic of Georgia, and Iraq. Before being injured, he was an expert licensed skydiver with over 1500 jumps and participated with a canopy formation team that set several world records in one weekend in 2004. He is highly decorated, with his top honor being the Legion of Merit. He is a member of the VFW in Hampton, VA, where he values the camaraderie of fellow veterans. His primary caregiver is his wonderful wife, Van (Vivian).

Printed in Great Britain
by Amazon

59384785R00096